QUALITY ASSURANCE IN DIAGNOSTIC RADIOLOGY

Quality Assurance in Diagnostic Radiology

A Guide Prepared Following a Workshop Held in Neuherberg,
Federal Republic of Germany, 20–24 October 1980,
and Organized Jointly by

Institute of Radiation Hygiene, Federal Health Office,
Neuherberg, Federal Republic of Germany

Society for Radiation and Environmental Research,
Neuherberg, Federal Republic of Germany

and

World Health Organization,
Geneva, Switzerland

WORLD HEALTH ORGANIZATION, GENEVA, 1982

ISBN 92 4 154164 4

TYPESET IN INDIA
PRINTED IN ENGLAND

81/5145–Macmillan/Procrom–6500

CONTENTS

CONTENTS

1. Introduction

A MEETING on efficacy and efficiency in the diagnostic application of radiation and radionuclides, held in Neuherberg in December 1979 by the organizers of the 1980 Workshop, concluded that an important step in the development of efficacy/efficiency studies would be the design and adoption by all countries of a programme of quality control and assurance in the domain of radiodiagnostic and nuclear medicine, with the aim of improving the diagnostic quality of procedures and reducing wastage. The meeting felt that WHO and the International Atomic Energy Agency should play a catalytic role in the design and implementation of this quality control and assurance programme. It also considered that better diagnostic images, which could lead to more accurate diagnoses and better-informed decisions regarding treatment, would benefit not only the health of individual patients but also the health status of the population—albeit that this effect is very difficult to demonstrate.

As a result of the above conclusions, a limited number of countries have initiated *quality assurance programmes*[1] in diagnostic radiology and nuclear medicine at the national level. However, in a greater number of countries such programmes are still only a local initiative and depend on the particular interest of specialists (radiologists, medical physicists, medical radiology technicians, etc.). Data gathered from 15 European countries using a WHO questionnaire show that *quality assurance*[1] in diagnostic radiology has entered national regulations in only a few countries.[2] The time now appears to be ripe for an international effort towards a more systematic approach in this field. The aim of the 1980 Workshop[3] (in which the United States Bureau of Radiological Health contributed technical support) was to gather together specialists with different backgrounds—diagnostic radiologists and medical

---

[1]For definitions of these terms, see Annex 1.

[2]In developing countries—despite the great limitation of resources—very little has been done to introduce quality assurance activities.

[3]Another international meeting—on quality assurance in nuclear medicine—was held in November 1980. A guide on this subject has been published by WHO as a companion volume to the present publication.

physicists, representatives of international organizations connected with diagnostic radiology, and a representative of the United States Bureau of Radiological Health with several years' experience in organizing quality assurance programmes at a national level—in order to effect an exchange of views on the work being carried out in a number of countries and the current activities of various international bodies. The main purpose of this exchange of experience was to provide some solid recommendations to be applied at the international, national, and radiodiagnostic department levels.

The present guide endeavours to provide an outline of the type of quality assurance programme to be recommended for (1) routine implementation by those performing radiodiagnostic procedures (medical radiology technicians, medical physicists, and radiologists), (2) for application by the responsible national authorities, and (3) for use by international bodies such as the International Society of Radiology (ISR), the International Commission on Radiological Protection (ICRP), and the International Commission on Radiation Units and Measurements (ICRU).

It is worth mentioning in this context that in redrafting one of its publications (25) ICRP has already mentioned the important role of quality assurance and the problem represented by the retake rate. At its meeting in July 1980, ICRU decided to establish five new report committees, of which three will deal respectively with:

—quality assurance of diagnostic radiological equipment;
—quality assurance of external beam radiotherapy; and
—specifications and quality assurance of scintillation cameras.

This accrued interest in quality assurance in diagnostic radiology emphasizes the urgent need for realistic recommendations and explicit programmes in this area, and for their prompt implementation throughout the world.

When quality assurance programmes are envisaged, three objectives are usually considered:
—cost containment;
—reduction in radiation exposure; and
—improvement of medical imaging.

Although quality assurance is only one of the possible approaches for reaching the above objectives, its role is important and merits greater attention than that at present given in the majority of countries.

The former United States Department of Health, Education, and Welfare[1] estimated the cost of diagnostic imaging services at US $7800 million per year. If the Department's estimated retake rate of approximately 6% (13) is accepted as valid, it could be argued that US $470 million are wasted on images of nondiagnostic quality. Although some retakes cannot be avoided, if a quality assurance programme led to even a 50% reduction of the retake rate, a saving of US $235 million could be expected from such a programme, which might involve the investment of only a relatively small sum.

---

[1]Renamed the United States Department of Health and Human Services in 1980.

In addition to the reduction in film wastage resulting from quality assurance, there is the further advantage of reducing patient and radiological personnel exposure, which (although not easy to quantify) can be expressed in grays and/or sieverts.

It should be stressed that less than 30 % of the world's population is endowed with well-developed health care services, including good radiodiagnostic coverage. In this guide, consideration has therefore been given to some simple approaches that could be implemented in countries in which the present situation is unsatisfactory and in which the need for quality assurance—though it might not seem so immediately obvious—is, in fact, much greater and more basic than in other parts of the world.

2. Aims of quality assurance in diagnostic radiology

THE provision of high-quality health care is the goal of all medical services. In the case of *diagnostic radiological facilities*,[1] patient selection, the conduct of the examination, and the interpretation of the results can all have an impact on the achievement of this goal. With respect to the conduct of the examination, it has been increasingly recognized that quality assurance programmes directed at equipment and operator performance can be of great value in improving the diagnostic information content, reducing radiation exposure, reducing medical costs, and improving departmental management. Quality assurance programmes thus contribute to the provision of high-quality health care.

2.1 Identification of needs

Experience has drawn attention to the needs and potential benefits to be derived from the implementation of effective quality assurance programmes. Several studies have indicated that many diagnostic radiological facilities produce poor-quality images and give unnecessary radiation exposure. An early indication of the existence of these problems was revealed by a medical surveillance programme conducted in the USA by the National Institute for Occupational Safety and Health in association with the Department of Labor's Pneumoconiosis Compensation Program. Trout et al. (*49*) found that, despite the prescreening of facilities and readers, 44 % of the facilities participating in the first round of examinations had from 10 % to 40 % of their submitted radiographs rejected as being of inadequate quality for the diagnosis of pneumoconiosis. These inadequate images represented unproductive radiation exposure as well as unsatisfactory medical care. Some of the reasons for the inadequacy were related to poor equipment performance.

An evaluation of preauthorization dental radiographs submitted to Pennsylvania Blue Shield (a statewide medical insurance plan) in the USA

---

[1] For a definition of this term, see Annex 1.

found that approximately 20% were unsatisfactory for reasons probably related to poor equipment performance (5).

A study of a number of general radiography facilities by the Du Pont Company (Delaware, USA) revealed that, on average, 13% of the radiographs processed were rejected as being of inadequate quality (16). An average of 9% of the radiographs taken had to be repeated. An analysis of the reasons for these rejections led to the conclusion that poor equipment performance was an important problem.

These three studies indicated that poor equipment performance made a significant contribution to the high prevalence of poor image quality. This finding is supported by the results of other studies, which have shown that electrical or mechanical problems may affect the performance of a large percentage of X-ray units (7, 43, 44).

The effect of poor-quality images is twofold. Obviously the radiologist would prefer to study an optimum-quality image even though he or she might be able to draw some useful conclusions from a poor image. If the image is not of adequate quality, practitioners may not have all the possible diagnostic information that could have been made available to them, and this may lead to an incorrect diagnosis. In addition, if the quality of the radiograph is so poor that it cannot be used, then the patient will have been unproductively exposed to radiation, causing an increase in the cost of diagnosis.

Unnecessary radiation exposure may also occur in the production of adequate-quality radiographs. Data from the Nationwide Evaluation of X-ray Trends (NEXT) programme, administered by the United States Bureau of Radiological Health, revealed that the "standard patient" (as defined in reference 37) can receive widely different exposures depending on the facility (or even on the machine within a facility) performing the examination (9). Even when a consideration of the NEXT data is limited, for example, to exposures by machines with a nominal peak tube potential of 80 kVp and half-value layers (HVL) of 2.5 mm of aluminium, the output at 30 cm varied from less than 12.9×10^{-7} C/kg to 258×10^{-7} C/kg when a current of one milliampere was applied for one second (9). Similar variations have been found in studies carried out in other countries (2, 20). The United States Bureau of Radiological Health has also studied the impact of the choice of image receptor on the exposure variation. Statistical analysis of the posterior/anterior (P/A) chest projection data has been carried out using the factors of kVp, HVL, relative speed of the image receptor, grid, type of processing, and $C.kg^{-1}$. It was found that these factors can account for only 50% of the exposure variation (41). In the Bureau of Radiological Health's view, machine malfunction causing the actual kVp and $C.kg^{-1}$ to deviate from the machine settings selected by the practitioner is a major cause of this variation. Such machine malfunction can be greatly reduced by effective quality assurance programmes.

A survey of the numbers and causes of spoilt X-ray films, which was carried out under the aegis of the Radiation Protection Committee of the British Institute of Radiology (6), revealed that exposure faults in 47% of the cases were the major reason for retakes—particularly in films taken with portable radiographic equipment. Malpositioning was shown to be the second major cause of retakes (25 %).

In 1980 a study was conducted (52) at a district hospital near Nairobi, Kenya, to evaluate the image quality of 50 X-ray films of the skull taken in both P/A and lateral positions: 20 % of the P/A views and 34 % of the lateral views were considered poor. Fogging and other reasons causing poor detail recognition were responsible for 50 % of the poor-quality P/A views, while 42 % of the poor-quality lateral views were attributable to malpositioning.

According to an Australian study (33), positioning errors were the major cause of film wastage—ranging from 8.8 % to 13.0 % for different film sizes. Also, there was a higher frequency of positioning errors in trauma patients. Exposure faults came second and equipment malperformance came third. There is no doubt that radiographic errors as well as poor equipment performance can contribute significantly to the need for retakes.

Thus several studies have identified problems of poor image quality and unnecessary radiation exposure in diagnostic radiological facilities. A more complete description of such findings has been published by the United States Bureau of Radiological Health (10). Quality assurance programmes directed at the equipment and its use are expected to have a major impact on reducing these problems.

2.2 Solution to the problem

A quality assurance programme may be defined as an organized effort by the staff operating a facility to ensure that the diagnostic images produced by the facility are of sufficiently high quality so that they consistently provide adequate diagnostic information at the lowest possible cost and with the least possible exposure of the patient to radiation. In its most comprehensive form, the quality assurance programme monitors each phase of operation of the diagnostic radiological facility, beginning with the request for an examination and ending with the interpretation of the examination and the communication of this interpretation to the referring physician. Included within this programme are actions to ensure that the radiology equipment used for the examination will yield the information desired about the patient. The actions considered in this guide include appropriate selection of equipment, as well as monitoring and maintenance of its performance.

Quality assurance programmes, designed to ensure that the radiology equipment can yield the desired information, include both *quality control*[1] techniques and *quality administration procedures*.[1] Quality control techniques are used to test the components of the radiological system to verify that the equipment is operating satisfactorily. Quality administration procedures encompass management actions designed to verify that the quality control monitoring techniques are performed regularly and properly, that the results

---

[1] For definitions of these terms, see Annex 1.

of these techniques are evaluated promptly and accurately, and that the necessary corrective measures are taken in response to these results. Quality administration procedures include the assignment of responsibility for quality assurance actions, the establishment of standards of quality for equipment in the facility, the provision of adequate training, and the selection of the appropriate equipment for each examination.

The question of the appropriateness of the equipment should be considered at the time it is ordered and installed. This involves a determination of the clinical imaging requirements for the equipment and the translation of these requirements into technical specifications, followed by the selection of equipment which satisfies the technical specifications, and finally the *acceptance inspection (acceptance test)*[1] of the equipment after installation to confirm that it actually performs at the level described in the technical specifications agreed upon by the manufacturer and the purchaser (*10, 17, 36*).

This approach to the equipment selection phase of a quality assurance programme for radiology equipment is outlined in Table 1. During the acceptance testing phase, performance data are compiled which serve as a comparative standard for similar data collected subsequently during routine quality control monitoring of the equipment as it is used diagnostically.

Table 1. Quality assurance in diagnostic radiology

Identification of imaging requirements	*Equipment*
Development of equipment specifications	*selection*
Selection of equipment	*phase*
Installation and acceptance testing of equipment	*Acceptance*
Release of equipment for clinical use	*phase*
Monitoring of equipment performance	*Quality control phase*

The quality control phase must be supported by quality administration procedures, which include the assignment of responsibility for monitoring and corrective actions and for the evaluation and review of the effectiveness of the overall quality assurance programme.

The fundamental responsibility for a quality assurance programme for any radiological facility must be placed upon the individual in charge of the facility. If the programme is to be successfully implemented, however, the responsibility for the routine quality control equipment monitoring phase must be delegated to the radiographers, who use the equipment on a day-to-day basis.

In facilities where they are available, physicists, radiology engineers, or specially trained quality control technicians should play a major role in the quality assurance programme. These specialized personnel may be assigned responsibility for the day-to-day administration of the programme and may

---

[1] For a definition of this term, see Annex 1.

carry out monitoring duties at a more advanced level. Responsibilities for certain quality control techniques and corrective measures may be assigned to personnel qualified by training and experience, such as consultants or industrial representatives from outside the facility.

Authorities at the state, federal, and international level can also play a key role in the implementation of effective quality control and assurance programmes.

3. Prerequisites for quality assurance programmes

RADIOLOGY imaging equipment should produce an image which meets the needs of the radiologist or other interpreters without involving unnecessary irradiation of the patient. Quality assurance actions contribute to the production of diagnostic images of a consistent quality by reducing the variations in performance of the imaging equipment. The quality control monitoring aspects of a quality assurance programme are, however, not necessarily related to the quality (information content) of the image. Prior to the initiation of a quality control monitoring programme, standards of acceptable image quality should be established. Ideally these standards should be objective—for example, acceptability limits for parameters that characterize image quality—but they may be subjective—for example, the opinions of professional personnel, in cases where adequate objective standards cannot be defined.

3.1 Retake analysis

A retake analysis (analysis of rejected films) is a subjective evaluation of image quality. Those images judged to be of inadequate quality are then categorized according to cause, which may be related to the competence of the technical personnel, equipment problems, specific difficulties associated with the examination, or some combination of these elements. A retake analysis also acts as a link between a department's quality assurance efforts and the consistency of its image quality.

As described in a comprehensive report on retakes by the United States Bureau of Radiological Health (13) retake analysis may be used: (a) to evaluate the problems leading to poor image quality; (b) as a self-improvement tool for the staff; and (c) as a management data base. In essence, the retake analysis provides an overall index of consistency related to image quality.

However, since the retake rate is established by the subjective evaluation of image quality, it is possible that a department may be approving the consistent production of images of poorer quality than those which could be achieved by the equipment. Constraints such as shortages of radiology personnel (particularly radiologists), lack of equipment maintenance and service, and logistic problems concerning X-ray films and chemicals are encountered by developing countries and may modify their approach to quality control. Only a few retake analyses have been recorded and these need to be interpreted in the light of the local conditions. At the University Hospital in Freetown, Sierra Leone, a total of 340 000 films per year are being analysed by two radiologists, and the retake rate recorded is 1 %. The Kenyatta Hospital in Nairobi rejects 5.9 % of all films taken per year, though the number of films analysed per radiologist per year is only about 40 % of that recorded for Sierra Leone. The wide range of different local circumstances, which influence the introduction of a retake analysis programme, as well as subjective criteria, on which the evaluation of retakes are based, make it difficult to draw comparisons between one facility and another.

An ongoing retake analysis programme should be coupled with a more objective evaluation of image quality in order to establish first of all the optimum level of image quality, bearing in mind the need to minimize patient exposure.

The most objective evaluation of image quality is the physical measurement of parameters, such as contrast, sharpness, modulation transfer function, and noise power spectrum. The determination of these physical quantities requires complex physical measurements which are beyond the scope of most departments of diagnostic radiology. Also, the relationship between the physical measurements and reader performance is often not well understood. Three alternatives to physical methods are discussed below. These methods vary in both complexity and the degree of "subjectiveness".

3.1.1 Radiologists' impressions

The most common method of image quality evaluation practised in diagnostic radiology departments is the evaluation of patient radiographs and fluoroscopic images by the radiologist. The performance of such evaluations is a routine part of the radiologist's responsibilities in the department and, as such, the results are seldom published in the literature. The evaluations are usually performed informally, without regard for statistical principles. This informal method is used, for example, to compare screen/film systems and scatter reduction techniques, or perhaps to establish optimum conditions for a new X-ray generator.

For example, a radiologist wishing to compare two screen/film systems, A and B, might either take two groups of patients and radiograph half the patients using system A and the other half using B, or take one group of patients and radiograph each individual twice, once with each system. The resultant radiographs would then be evaluated and compared by the radiologist applying subjective criteria, and the system which in his opinion produced the higher-quality images would be judged to be the better of the two for the particular application tested.

To the radiologist this is a practical, common-sense way of quickly evaluating image quality. However, it induces a false sense of security, since— although the radiologist is confident of his own decision—there is no correct answer against which the decision may be checked, and, because it was based on results that are not quantifiable or amenable to analysis, it could lead to false conclusions. The establishment of internationally accepted criteria for diagnostic image quality should therefore be considered as an important future goal.

3.1.2 *Visibility of anatomical landmarks*

An alternative to the previous method of image evaluation is for the radiologist to judge the visibility of predefined anatomical landmarks in a series of images selected for evaluation (*50*). This method has been successfully utilized in several statistically acceptable clinical evaluations without over-burdening the department's staff (*19, 40, 42, 45, 48, 51*). It is based on the assumption that the quality of visualization of anatomical landmarks is directly related to that of significant radiographic details. Specific anatomical landmarks were chosen as criteria because of their relationship to the radiographic manifestation of disease or trauma. It is reasonable to assume that if these landmarks are well visualized on a radiograph, then the radiograph is capable of displaying most details of pathological interest. Some exceptions occur, but the technique has been found to be useful in many clinical applications.

The use of anatomical criteria to evaluate radiographic images straddles the gap between the radiologist's subjective impressions of image quality and the results of physical measurements. The use of this method in conjunction with physical evaluations of radiographic images facilitates correlation of the radiologist's subjective evaluations of image quality with the physical parameters used to characterize the image.

Compared with the radiologist's subjective impressions of image quality, the use of anatomical criteria is more difficult to implement in a clinical setting. In order to achieve more objective and scientifically rigorous results than those deriving from the radiologist's impressions, this method requires careful statistical design, randomized selection of patients, a high degree of quality control during the production of the test images, and single-blind evaluation. Furthermore, the results from the use of anatomical criteria allow a level of analysis that provides an understanding of the effects of image quality on the visibility of particular organ systems or specific anatomical details of importance.

There are other features of the use of anatomical criteria for image evaluation that make it particularly suitable for diagnostic radiological facilities. No special equipment is required to perform the evaluation and the results obtained are directly related to patient images and clinical ap-plications—in fact the results can be confined to a particular examination or task.

3.1.3 *Observer performance*

Another method of image evaluation available to radiological facilities, which is highly task specific, is the measurement of observer performance.

Observer performance, as judged by the determination of the presence or absence of a signal, can be used to compare the quality of clinical imaging systems. The bias of a single observer is overcome by the use of several observers and multiple sample images.

The Receiver Operating Characteristic (ROC) curve is the conventional method for displaying the results of observer performance studies (*34, 35, 46, 47*). It has come into use because it offers several advantages over other indices of performance that have been proposed. ROC analysis describes the ability of both the observer(s) and the equipment to detect the signal in a way which takes into account the confidence level used by the observer to decide if a signal is present. This confidence level is one of the parameters of the curve— strict, moderate, or lax criteria. ROC analysis is also independent of the signal's occurrence in the sample population.

Observer performance studies employing ROC analysis for image evaluation are more difficult to conduct than the "common-sense" method or the application of anatomical criteria to image evaluation. Observer performance studies require a statistically significant sample of cases in which the correct diagnosis is known, if ROC analysis is to be performed. Verification of cases for such a sample is usually quite time-consuming. However, the strength of ROC analysis is that it can provide a highly objective comparison of the performance of the imaging systems for the applications considered. Since the results are specific to the imaging task, caution must be used when generalizing the conclusions to broader applications.

3.2 Test objects

The use of test objects supplements the retake analysis of patient radiographs in evaluating image quality and equipment performance. Two types of test objects are used to evaluate image quality in radiology departments—anthropomorphic and physical. Anthropomorphic test objects are constructed to mimic the radiographic appearance of the body part or anatomical region of interest. Physical test objects are so constructed that their radiographic interpretation or measurement is related to physical parameters of interest.

Anthropomorphic test objects are used to compare the image quality between different radiographic imaging systems or after modifications to a given system. The comparison can be strictly subjective, in the manner of the "common-sense" method described earlier (see section 3.1.1). In this case, the phantom is radiographed on each of the radiographic systems being evaluated and the image quality is assessed subjectively according to the reader's impression of these radiographs (*12*).

Anthropomorphic phantoms can also be used in conjunction with anatomical criteria (*11, 51*) and, in addition, are useful in evaluating fluoroscopic systems.

The advantages of the anthropomorphic test objects for image evaluation are largely derived from their permanent construction. Unlike patients, there is no inherent variability from image to image. Anthropomorphic phantoms can be used to produce a large sample size of images under controlled conditions, and in observer performance studies the true positives and false positives can be known absolutely. Also, the use of anthropomorphic phantoms obviates the necessary consideration of the ethics associated with the use of human subjects. The disadvantage is that no single phantom can mimic patient-to-patient variation, nor can the signals introduced represent true pathology. There is also the uncertain impact on image quality of physiological motion, a factor not present in an anthropomorphic phantom. The absence of motion could lead to erroneous conclusions (*11, 51*). Therefore, anthropomorphic phantoms are probably best used as a first-line evaluation tool to rule out any inappropriate radiographic systems.

In addition, physical test objects are also used to evaluate image quality in radiology departments. With the exception of the common step-wedge, which displays dynamic range, physical test objects fall into two categories. The first category of test objects is used to evaluate high-contrast resolution and includes bar patterns, star patterns, wire meshes, and thin wires made from relatively high radio-opaque materials. The second category is used to evaluate low-contrast perceptibility with examples such as arrays of holes of varying depth in plastic blocks, plastic spheres, and discs. For both categories evaluation is performed by recording the minimum visible signal produced under the imaging conditions being evaluated.

3.3 Conclusions

The previous sections discussed means of evaluating image quality. To ensure that the facility is consistent in its evaluations it is recommended that standards of acceptable image quality should be defined during the establishment of a quality assurance programme. These standards would express the amount of variation in equipment performance which the facility feels it can tolerate while still maintaining acceptable image quality and minimizing radiation exposure. Not all fluctuations are serious enough to cause image quality problems. Therefore, to attempt to ensure perfectly stable equipment performance would be both fruitless and expensive. Standards for image quality help the staff of the facility to decide when the detected variations in performance are serious enough to require corrective action.

Ideally these standards should be objective. For example, the standard of quality related to processor performance might be stated in terms of the acceptable range of optical densities found through sensitometric monitoring of the processor. Since variations greater than this range may lead to poor image quality, they would call for corrective action. It is recognized, however, that for many parameters of the diagnostic radiological system, the standards of image quality will remain partially subjective for some time to come. This is largely because of a lack of consensus among medical practitioners as to what constitutes "good" quality; and also it is still not clear what impact variations in some parameters have on image quality. Practitioners in each facility are encouraged to establish their own standards of image quality based on their training and experience, using methods such as those described in this chapter, and to relate these standards to measures of system performance.

4. Organizational framework

QUALITY assurance programmes at the facility level may be influenced by several major entities (Fig. 1). These entities are both internal or external to the diagnostic facility. It is obvious that interactions other than those indicated in Fig. 1 are possible.

Fig. 1. Major entities influencing quality assurance programmes at the facility level

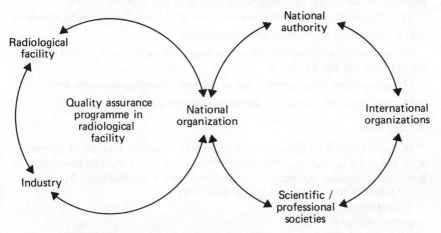

Three elements are usually involved with the implementation of a quality assurance programme in a diagnostic facility:

(1) the radiological facility staff—physicians, physicists, radiographers;

(2) the manufacturer; and

(3) the national organizations—governmental, medical physics, and physicians groups.

Organizations at the national level normally work in association with governmental authorities at the national and international levels and with professional societies and organizations.

On an international level, various bodies—such as WHO, Commission of the European Communities (CEC), International Commission on Radiological Protection (ICRP), International Commission on Radiation Units and Measurements (ICRU), International Electrotechnical Commission (IEC), International Organization of Medical Physicists (IOMP), International Organization for Standardization (ISO), International Radiation Protection Association (IRPA), and International Society of Radiology (ISR)—may interact with either the national authorities or the professional societies, or both.

In the following sections, some details are given of the ways in which each of these entities influences the quality assurance programme.

4.1 Essential elements of a quality assurance programme

4.1.1 Criteria and test methods

Criteria and test methods must be established. These may be developed at the international level, at a national level (by regulations, codes of practice, and/or recommendations), or at a local level (within the radiological facility). In the last case, extra requirements may be incorporated into the purchase contract between the radiological facility and the manufacturers.

The criteria should include consideration of at least the following elements:

(1) identification of imaging requirements;

(2) performance characteristics of radiological equipment related to image quality and patient exposure;

(3) acceptance requirements for newly purchased equipment; and

(4) radiation protection of patients and workers.

4.1.2 Testing

In order to verify whether or not the relevant parameters are in agreement with the criteria, test measurements must be carried out. The measurement techniques should be simple to perform and reproducible. Appropriate consideration must be given to the following:
—instruments,
—personnel, and
—protocols, for data collection and recording.

4.1.3 Interpretation of results, feedback, and record-keeping

Analysis of the results should be a continuous process, so that, in case of discrepancy between the results and the requirements, appropriate action can be taken to bring the performance characteristics back to the required level (feedback). Thorough record-keeping of all results, analyses, and corrective actions is highly recommended because this may help to disclose hidden problems.

4.1.4 *Further elements*

A suitable organizational structure should be established to facilitate all actions taken in the context of the quality assurance programme and to assure benefit from them. It should include the following elements:

(1) assignment of responsibilities;

(2) establishment of a quality assurance committee;

(3) time schedules for the monitoring and maintenance of radiological equipment;

(4) maintenance of test equipment;

(5) record-keeping and reporting;

(6) budgetary provisions; and

(7) training of personnel.

In carrying out a quality assurance programme the radiological facility may need the support and advisory service of various organizations outside the facility:

—scientific/professional societies (national or international),

—national organization(s),

—national authorities,

—international bodies, and

—manufacturers.

4.2 Organization within the radiological facility

4.2.1 *Personnel requirements*

The person in charge of the facility should have primary responsibility for implementing and maintaining the quality assurance programme. Normally, the radiographer will be delegated a primary quality assurance role by the physician in charge. In the past, a great deal of emphasis has been placed on the need for adequate medical physics input in radiation therapy, although, in the area of radiodiagnosis, a similar level of attention to the needs and availability of an adequate medical physics input has not generally been considered necessary. Recent studies have, however, demonstrated that the problems in the area of diagnostic radiology justify the assistance of physicists/engineers. The development of an understanding of the scientific basis of cost–risk–benefit analysis by physicists has resulted in both a reduction of patient and staff exposure doses and an improvement in diagnostic efficiency and financial savings. For the adequate organization and execution of a quality assurance programme, it is of key importance for the radiological facility to have access to and make use of radiophysics services with expertise in this field. These services may involve not only scientific knowledge and technical expertise, but also special equipment and/or personnel.

In the absence of nearby radiophysics services, it may be necessary to obtain the expertise through contact with other hospitals, institutions, governmental or other organizations, or industry.

The training of all personnel involved is an important element in any quality assurance programme.

4.2.2 *The planning of a quality assurance programme*

When a quality assurance programme is implemented in a radiological facility, basic tests must be distinguished from routine tests.

If a radiological facility cannot carry out its own quality assurance programme and relies on outside support, an appropriate contract should be made with the supporting organization. A radiological facility can implement its own quality assurance programme only if sufficient instrumentation and manpower are available.

A periodic review of a facility's quality assurance programme by the physician in charge, or by the quality assurance committee, should look for any shortcomings or possible improvements.

4.2.3 *Measurements within the quality assurance programme*

(1) *Baseline measurements*

When a quality assurance programme is initiated, it is highly desirable to establish the baseline level of performance of radiology equipment by fully assessing the specified performance characteristics. A record of these will then serve as a reference against which the future performance of the equipment can be compared.

Such a comprehensive assessment should also be carried out on all new equipment. It needs to be repeated when (*a*) routine checks indicate a specified deviation in performance, (*b*) after major maintenance, and (*c*) after any modifications to parts of the equipment that affect performance characteristics.

(2) *Routine checks*

It is essential that simple and speedy routine checks should be carried out to provide assurance that the radiology equipment continues to perform satisfactorily.

These checks should be regularly repeated, at a frequency determined by the probability of malfunction of the equipment under test. Results of routine checks should be recorded in an equipment log-book.

In cases in which it has not been possible to establish the baseline level of performance to the extent described in paragraph (1) above, it has been demonstrated that certain routine checks have still proved to be of value.

The correct performance of appropriately calibrated test equipment used in quality assurance programmes needs to be routinely checked and recorded.

4.2.4 *Analysis of measurements and checks*

Any analysis of the results of a quality assurance programme needs to be made by a competent and experienced person. After considering both the standards of acceptable image quality and the errors inherent in the quality assurance measurements, this analysis should determine whether the performance is acceptable and, if not, what corrective actions should be taken.

4.3 Equipment manufacture

Diagnostic X-ray units should be manufactured so as to comply with the performance characteristics included in the latest national and international guidelines and recommendations; they should also meet any special requirements agreed upon between manufacturer and customer. The manufacturer should provide a signed document specifying the performance characteristics of a unit, and the radiological facility should not formally receive equipment until acceptance tests have verified that these specifications have been met. (It will sometimes be desirable for the manufacturer to assist in making these acceptance tests.)

4.4 The national organization

The implementation of a quality assurance programme will be aided if an organization at the national level carries out the following tasks:

(1) providing assistance and coordination in setting up local quality assurance programmes;

(2) performing the entire quality assurance programme, or a specific part of it, in a radiological facility, in order to compensate for any deficiencies that may exist in local capabilities or competence (especially in acceptance tests);

(3) ascertaining, on a selective basis, the adequacy of quality assurance programmes, and advising accordingly;

(4) developing and/or disseminating recommendations, codes of practice, regulations, requirements, norms, etc., generated by national authorities, international bodies, and professional societies;

(5) ensuring the provision of calibration facilities for the test equipment used in any local quality assurance programme; and

(6) helping to analyse the results of quality assurance programmes, and finding technical solutions to improve performance characteristics.

4.5 Scientific/professional societies

Scientific/professional societies are expected to collaborate in the implementation of quality assurance programmes. Their role can be the following:

(1) to promote the concepts of quality assurance in scientific meetings;

(2) to collaborate with the national organization so that this organization is able to do its work in the radiological facility;

(3) to participate in training activities; and

(4) to provide guidelines, etc. (either directly to the radiological facility or through the national organization).

4.6 National authorities

The national authorities could be involved in appropriate legislative measures which would support the tasks of the national organization, as described in section 4.4.

4.7 International bodies

The role of international bodies tends to be restricted to providing general recommendations in order to encourage countries to adopt certain activities and to coordinate those activities.

International bodies (see page 22) could play a catalytic role in the design and implementation of quality assurance programmes. Their activities might include such functions as:

—intercomparison of quality assurance programmes at the international level;

—organization of international meetings, seminars, workshops, etc.; and

—publication of guidelines and recommendations relating to the performance characteristics of diagnostic X-ray equipment.

5. Specific equipment considerations

5.1 General aspects

SECTIONS 5.2–5.6 provide information and instruction on the technical aspects involved in a quality assurance programme. The performance parameters to be controlled range from simple to highly sophisticated, in an effort to meet the requirements of small one-room facilities as well as those of more sophisticated radiodiagnostic departments. When planning to implement a quality assurance programme, each facility, regardless of its size or level of sophistication, should take into consideration the following general aspects.

It is advisable to establish minimum levels of performance, below which the equipment should not continue to be used. Also, different criteria may need to be applied, depending on the use and type of equipment. Minimum levels of equipment performance will probably differ from the levels of acceptable performance applicable to new installations.

The most important objectives of a quality assurance programme comprise:

(1) detection of defects on installation, or after major repair, that may adversely affect image quality or patient dose;

(2) establishment of a baseline of performance against which future measurements can be compared and maintenance of the original level of acceptable performance can be confirmed.

(3) assistance in detecting and diagnosing the cause of any deterioration in performance;

(4) correction of any deterioration in performance when the cause is known; and

(5) assistance in enabling comparable X-ray exposure factors to be used on different X-ray machines where appropriate.

All test methods must be performed in accordance with nationally and internationally established safe working procedures. No invasive test methods should be attempted without the manufacturer's cooperation or approval, in order to avoid invalidation of warranties. Whenever possible, routine tests should exclude invasive methods.

For a facility which has not yet performed quality control tests, a step-by-step implementation of a quality assurance programme is recommended. This should start with baseline measurements (e.g., retake analysis) and simple routine tests (e.g., processor performance).

Sections 5.2–5.5 contain tables which give a condensed overview of the subjects dealt with in the text. Notes are added, indicating the most suitable person(s) to carry out each test, the priority given to each parameter, and the recommended frequency of testing. However, flexibility should be allowed in deciding who should carry out the tests in a particular facility. In some facilities, a highly trained radiographer or technician could carry out tests normally allocated to a physicist; whereas in other facilities, a physicist or engineer may be needed for the satisfactory performance of tests normally assigned to a radiographer.

It is often convenient and cost-effective to use simple methods to check the overall performance of a facility's radiographic, fluoroscopic, and other systems. This can be simply performed by employing a suitable phantom under standard conditions. Specific and sophisticated methods should be used only when indicated.

It is desirable that each facility should have the possibility of performing the tests listed as essential. Cost–benefit considerations will have an impact on the frequency of the quality control procedures, apart from the guidelines given in the text.

5.2 Radiographic equipment: parameters to be checked (Table 2)

5.2.1 The generator and control system

(1) *The kVp applied* to the X-ray tube should be checked to ensure that it is in reasonable agreement with the kVp indicated on the control panel. The direct measurement of kVp is not practicable as a routine test. The most common indirect method is to determine the peak voltage from measurements of radiation quality. The photometric filter method is easy to use if a suitable calibrated penetrameter is available (*3, 32*).

Tests will usually need to be carried out at various values of kVp and tube current; with some types of penetrameter it may be necessary to use two instruments to cover a wide range of X-ray tube voltages.

(2) *The radiation output* should be measured at a set distance (conventionally 75 cm or 1 m) and expressed in units such as C/kg per mA.s applied to the tube. The values obtained should be checked against published data (*23–25, 38*). They will need to be measured over a range of voltages and with different tube currents. On installation, and after major repair, it will be necessary for a physicist to carry out this measurement with a calibrated dosimeter, but routine tests to check whether the output has changed can be performed by a radiographer—if a simple dosimeter is available (*15*).

(3) *The exposure timing device* should be checked. This can often be done with either a spinning top (preferably electrically driven) or a simple electronic

Table 2.   Parameters to be checked on radiographic equipment

Recom- mended priority[a]	Text section No.	Item	Personnel category[b]	on instal- lation	after repair	as necess- rary	W[c]	D[c]
A	5.2.1	Tube potential (kV$_p$)	P/R	X	X	X		
A		Automatic expo- sure system	P	X		X		
A		Filtration	P	X	X			
A		Removable filters	R					X
A	5.2.2	Light localizer	P/R	X	X	X		
A		Grids	R	X	X	X		
A		Mechanical stability	R	X				X
B		Radiation output	P/R	X	X	X	X	
B	5.2.1	Timer	P/R	X		X		
B	5.2.1	Controls	P/R	X				
C		Meter zero	R				X	
C	5.2.2	Couch top absorption	P	X	X			
B	5.2.1	Area exposure	P	X	X			
B	5.2.2	Focal spot size	P	X	X			

KEY: [a] A = essential; B = necessary for good practice; C = important.
  [b] P = physicist or engineer; R = radiographer or technician.
  [c] W = weeky; D = daily (or more frequently, as necessary).

timer (8). Consistency of performance is essential—proportionality between the set time and the actual irradiation time is more important than the accuracy of the time measurement. With the exception of a falling-load generator, there should also be proportionality between exposure time and radiation output. It is important not only to establish the minimum exposure times that can be obtained consistently, but also to establish that the timing device reliably terminates the exposure, over the whole range of possible exposure times. Where an automatic exposure system is in use, it may be convenient to establish consistency by using a suitable dosimeter. Again, checks on the shortest practicable exposure times will be necessary (44).

(4) Where an *area exposure product meter* is fitted to an X-ray tube used for radiography, appropriate checks on its performance are necessary (30).

(5) *All controls should be clearly labelled.* Where X-ray equipment labelling is not clear enough to enable someone new to the equipment to select the correct tube, accessories, and operating conditions quickly and with certainty, the user should supplement the manufacturer's labels with additional, explicit, labels.

(6) At frequent intervals, checks should be made to see that all *electrical meters* are correctly set at zero, and adjusted as necessary. The meter should give an appropriate reading when the controls are set suitably.

5.2.2 *The X-ray tube, housing, and stand*

(1) It is essential that *total filtration* should conform to national or international (ICRP) standards. While it is often quite simple to check the thickness of added filtration, it is usually difficult to check the inherent filtration. The total filtration can be checked most easily by measuring the half-value layer of the radiation at given values of X-ray tube voltage, and comparing the results with published tables (such as those given in reference *24*). When interchangeable filters are available for special investigations, it is essential that a method should be devised to enable the operator to become immediately aware of the fact, in the event that they are not restored to normal.

(2) Checks on the *accuracy of visual delineation* of the X-ray beam can be carried out using a fluorescent screen with adequate shielding, but a method using a radiographic film is preferable. At one metre from the focal spot, the indication should be correct to within a centimetre on all four edges, and this should be maintained for any direction in which the beam may be used. Further, when the angular and other scales indicate that the beam is centered to any particular position (e.g., the centre line of the couch top or the chest stand), this, too, should be correct to within one centimetre at one metre from the focal spot. Where a small beam is checked on a large film, the presence of large amounts of off-focus radiation can often be detected. However, a similar film, overexposed during the beam adjustment test, will show much smaller amounts of off-focus radiation, because when a large aperture is used, off-focus radiation is more difficult to detect.

(3) Where an *antiscatter grid* is incorporated into the X-ray equipment, tests should be made to check that it is uniform, is installed perpendicularly to the beam, is correctly centered and remains so, and is designed for the required distance.

A test film exposed through the grid should not show appreciable density trends across the film.

(4) Any sign of *mechanical instability or malfunction* should be corrected immediately. Items to be noted include the efficiency of brakes and locks, correct indication of angular scales, rigidity of tube stand, etc.: the checking of these is particularly important on mobile and portable equipment, which may not always be used on a level floor.

(5) When a *couch top or other patient support* is replaced, checks should be made to ensure that if the radiation absorption of the replacement differs significantly from that of the previous support, the radiographic exposure factors are amended accordingly.

(6) The measurement of *focal spot size* is difficult, but two methods are available (*23*). In view of the role occupied by this factor in determining

resolution, it may be preferable to carry out this measurement on installation, to provide a baseline for later checking.

5.3 Image recording and processing equipment: parameters to be checked (Table 3)

5.3.1 Films

Checks need to be made to ensure that arrangements for film transport and storage (both before and after use) are such as to minimize deleterious effects. Boxes should be stored vertically on slat-type shelves in a well-ventilated store, free from X-radiation and fumes, preferably at 10–18 °C and a relative humidity of less than 50%. They should be used in strict chronological rotation. After use, films should be carefully filed for rapid recall.

5.3.2 Cassettes

(1) Each cassette should be marked to indicate the type of intensifying screen it contains and whether or not it is lead-backed.

(2) One intensifying screen in each cassette should be marked at the edge, so that it is possible to identify which cassette was used in the exposure of any particular film.

(3) Cassettes should be checked to ensure that there is uniformity of compression over the area of the screens. This can be accomplished most easily by radiographing a suitable test object—for example, a perforated grid in close contact with the front of the cassette (4).

(4) Intensifying screens should be examined for contamination or damage, and cleaned as necessary. Examination under ultraviolet radiation will often reveal things undetectable by ordinary light, as will a low exposure radiograph.

(5) Occasionally all cassettes in a particular X-ray facility should be exposed to a given dose of radiation, so that intercassette variations in speed can be detected.

(6) Each film processed should be checked for evidence of leakage of light into the cassette by looking for dark patches on the edges of the film.

5.3.3 Daylight loading systems

Any tendency for a daylight loading system to deliver two films at once, or none at all, requires immediate checking and adjustment or replacement.

5.3.4 Film processing

(1) *General matters:*
(a) Checks should be made to ensure that the safelight system is satisfactory. Such tests should use X-ray film, pre-exposed to give a density somewhat above the threshold, and then partially exposed to the safelight.

Table 3. Parameters to be checked on radiographic image recording and processing equipment

Recommended priority[a]	Text section No.	Item	Personnel category[b]	on installation	after repair	as necessary	A[c]	D[c]
		Cassettes and screens						
A		Light tightness	R			X	X	
A		Uniformity of compression	R			X	X	
A		Labelling screen type	R	X	X			
B	5.3.2	Labelling of lead backing	R	X	X			
B		Screen surface condition	R			X		
B		Screen identification	R	X	X			
B		Screen speed	P/R				X	
B	5.3.3	*Daylight loading systems*	R					
		General processing						
A		Selection of chemicals	R	X	X			
B		Identification markers	R					
B		Replenishment	R			X		
	5.3.4	*Manual processing*						
A		Developer temperature	R					
B		Fixing	R					
B		Adequate washing	R					
B		Tank cleaning	R			X		
		Automatic processing						
A		Sensitometric test	P/R					X
B	5.3.4	Water supplies	R					
B		Fixer pH	R					
B		Roller cleaning	R					

Table 3 (*continued*).

Recom-mended priority[a]	Text section No.	Item	Personnel category[b]	Testing required:				
				on instal-lation	after repair	as necess-ary	A[c]	D[c]
		Darkroom						
B	5.3.4	Room darkness	R	X	X			
B		Safelight	R	X		X		
		Viewing boxes						
B		Light uniformity	R	X		X		
B		Spotlight	R	X	X			
B	5.3.5	Tube replace-ment	R			X		
B		Blanking-off screen	R	X	X			
B		Screen uniformity	M	X				
B		Ambient light	M	X	X			

KEY: [a] A = essential; B = necessary for good practice.
   [b] P = Physicist or engineer; R = radiographer or technician; M = radiologist.
   [c] A = annually; D = daily (or more frequently, as necessary).

(b) Processing chemicals should be selected to match the emulsion(s) to be processed. They should be stored on shelves in a well-ventilated store, at $10-18°C$, and used in chronological rotation. They should be made up in a well-ventilated room in strict accordance with the manufacturer's instructions.

(c) Identification markers must be checked to ensure that they operate satisfactorily.

(d) Replenishment is necessary, and should be carried out strictly according to the manufacturer's instructions.

(2) *Manual processing:*

(a) A thermometer to indicate the developer temperature must always be observable.

(b) Whether or not the developer temperature is controlled thermostatically, it must be monitored, and developing times changed as appropriate.

(c) Film washing must be adequate (30 minutes in running water or the equivalent), and drying must be in a dust-free atmosphere.

(d) Fixing must be adequate. This requires the checking of the clearing time and the fixer pH.

(*e*) At a frequency dependent on the tank material, all tanks should be emptied and thoroughly cleaned according to the manufacturer's instructions.

(3) *Automatic processing:*

(*a*) Checks must be made to ensure that water supplies are at the appropriate temperature, and that the flow is adequate. This requires periodic checking of the filters.

(*b*) The mixing of different film types, or films from different manufacturers, in the same processor should only be carried out where tests have shown this to be satisfactory.

(*c*) Test strips should preferably be of the same X-ray film as that used clinically, and each test strip should (as far as possible) have received the same set of exposures (preferably using a light sensitometer) just prior to processing in order to avoid film-fading. It may be satisfactory to compare the test strips with a standard strip by eye. Where a densitometer is available, fog, contrast, and speed should be measured and then recorded to detect long-term trends. In general, all processors in a facility should give identical results. Any processor set up differently for a special purpose should be so marked. When new processors are first used in a facility, it is often advantageous to process one test strip at the same time every day. Very small random variations between one day and the next can usually be disregarded, since they may be due simply to temperature variations—moreover, it is often difficult to make small corrections to the operation of a processor. Persistent trends should be watched carefully. Experience will indicate when it is no longer necessary to carry out this procedure daily, but perhaps on alternate days or weekly. The fact that a test strip is different from that of the previous day does not necessarily indicate that there has been a change in the operation of the processor, although this is usually the most likely explanation. Other possible causes include change in film speed from batch to batch and faults in the X-ray generator.

(*d*) The fixer pH requires regular checking.

(*e*) It is important to ensure that the rollers are kept clean.

5.3.5 *Viewing boxes*

(1) The luminance of the viewing screen should not vary by more than 10% over the area of the film.

(2) When one fluorescent tube requires replacement, all the tubes in the viewing box, or set of viewing boxes, should be replaced at the same time.

(3) Within one facility, all viewing screens should use the same colour of fluorescent tube and have approximately the same brightness.

(4) A spotlight should be available as a part of, or adjacent to, every viewing box or set of viewing boxes.

(5) Blanking-off screens should be available.

(6) Ambient light should not be allowed to interfere with the diagnosis.

5.4 Fluoroscopic equipment: parameters to be checked (Table 4)

5.4.1 *Tube and generator performance*

Before any performance tests are undertaken on a fluoroscopic imaging system, it is advisable to check the performance of the X-ray tube and generator. This can be carried out in the manner described in sections 5.2.1 (1), (2), (4), (6), and 5.2.2 (1), (6), except that measurements of radiation output and checks on tube kilovoltage need to be performed under fluoroscopic operating conditions.

5.4.2 *Automatic exposure rate control*

In order to ensure that the patient receives the minimum radiation exposure necessary to produce an image of acceptable diagnostic quality, it is essential to check the correct functioning of the automatic exposure rate control. This is normally defined in terms of (*a*) the minimum and maximum levels of exposure rate at the input plane of the image intensifier, when the system operates under automatic control, and (*b*) the level obtained under typical operating conditions (*18, 21*).

The entrance dose rates in the patient may also be measured using an appropriate phantom, and with the fluoroscopic equipment operating as specified above.

It is also advisable to check that reductions in X-ray field size, by beam collimation, do not give rise to excessive increases in the levels of exposure rate at the intensifier when the equipment is operating under automatic control (i.e., increases should be no greater than 100%).

5.4.3 *Field size and distortion*

It is a relatively simple matter to check the field size and distortion of the intensifier–television system by means of a rectangular wire grid. Large differences in the observed and specified field sizes indicate that the system is not operating correctly. Alternatively, a considerable degree of distortion can usually be tolerated before the diagnostic information of the image is impaired (*18, 21, 27, 31*). In exceptional circumstances an unacceptable degree of "S-shaped" distortion may occur as a result of the influence of the earth's magnetic field on the imaging system.

5.4.4 *Beam collimation and alignment*

A fluorescent screen, together with adequate shielding, may be used to ascertain whether, under fluoroscopic operating conditions, the X-ray beam is confined to the area of the image receptor and is correctly centred (*18*). A similar check is necessary if the system incorporates a spot film device, since apparent errors in beam collimation and alignment may be due to the malfunctioning of the device.

If the system also includes an antiscatter grid, then this should also be checked, in the manner described in section 5.2.2 (3).

5.4.5 *Conversion factor*

An assessment should be made of the efficiency of the image receptor in converting X-rays to light. This involves a measurement of the luminance of the output fluorescent screen, using a calibrated photometer with a spectral sensitivity similar to that of the human eye under photopic conditions.

The conversion factor should be sufficient to ensure acceptable diagnostic image quality without excessive irradiation of the patient. Measurements should also be made at several points throughout the field of view in order to establish that no excessive variation exists, although some decrease at the edge of the field is to be expected (*21, 28, 29*).

5.4.6 *Contrast ratio/veiling glare*

The degree of "contrast loss" within the image intensifier should not be excessive. It is expressed using the concepts of contrast ratio or veiling glare (*32*) and is derived from a comparison of the measurements of a conversion factor in the centre of the field of view with and without a lead mask covering the central 10 % of the intensifier input area. A low value of contrast ratio may also arise in systems where a significant amount of off-focus radiation is generated.

5.4.7 *Grey scale test object for television monitor*

A test object capable of producing several steps of X-ray contrast, increasing linearly from 0 to 1.0, and also containing low contrast detail in areas of the image at high and low levels of brightness, may be used to ensure that the television monitor controls of brightness and contrast are set at optimum positions. The test object may then be used to confirm that an acceptable grey scale image with all the regular increments in contrast is visible (*22*).

It is advisable to perform this test before proceeding to carry out the tests described in sections 5.4.8, 5.4.9, and 5.4.10 below.

5.4.8 *Limiting resolution*

In order to check the limiting resolution of the system, the image of a lead bar test pattern may be observed under conditions of high contrast and low signal noise.

If the test pattern is small—compared with the field size—then additional measurements may be made throughout the field of view, in order to check the degree of uniformity of resolution (*18, 21*).

5.4.9 *Threshold contrast (noise)*

The images of large-size, low-contrast objects may be obscured by noise and contrast loss in the intensifier–television system. A test object containing details of this nature and of known contrast should be observed by utilizing X-ray beam qualities that are typical of normal fluoroscopic conditions (*21*).

5.4.10 *Minimum visible detail versus contrast test object*

A test object containing details covering a known wide range of sizes and levels of contrast may be used under standard exposure conditions to establish the variation in threshold contrast level that is just visible for each detail size, at specified exposure rates (*21*).

5.4.11 *Lag/afterglow*

It is advisable to assess the degree of lag or afterglow in the imaging system, because of the effect this may have on the visualization of dynamic images.

Further research is necessary to develop a test for this purpose that can be easily used in diagnostic facilities.

5.4.12 *General comments on test procedures*

(1) All the parameters described in in sections 5.4.1–5.4.11 above are relevant to the performance of both image intensifiers and light amplifiers associated with closed-circuit television systems.

(2) With regard to the performance of direct viewing systems, only sections 5.4.1, 5.4.4, 5.4.5, 5.4.8, 5.4.9, and 5.4.10 are relevant.

(3) It should be noted that, at the present stage of development, for the same level of patient dose, the image quality provided by image intensifier systems is superior to that of light amplifier systems, which in turn is superior to that of direct viewing systems.

(4) In the event of suspected malfunction of equipment, some of the checks described in sections 5.4.1–5.4.11 may be repeated with the image intensifier alone, after removal of the television camera. This serves to establish which part of the system is defective. However, before an attempt is made to remove the camera, attention should be paid to the comments in section 5.1 about invasive test methods.

(5) When measurements are taken immediately to the rear of intensifier systems from which the television camera has been removed, care must be exercised to avoid exposure to X-radiation passing out of the open end of the intensifier.

(6) All the parameters described in sections 5.4.1–5.4.11 should be checked by the physicist/engineer when new equipment is installed or when a quality assurance programme for old equipment is initiated.

(7) A routine check on the parameters described in sections 5.4.1, 5.4.2, 5.4.8, and 5.4.9 should be carried out at weekly intervals in order to ensure that the system performance has not deviated from the prescribed levels. This may be achieved by the radiographer's observing a single test object containing small detail of high contrast, large detail of low contrast, and appropriate beam filtration imaged under typical fluoroscopic conditions.

5.4.13 Operational factors relevant to fluoroscopic techniques

(1) Direct viewing fluoroscopy should never be undertaken unless the room is adequately darkened and the operator is adequately dark-adapted for at least 15 minutes beforehand.

(2) During image intensifier fluoroscopy, direct illumination of the television monitor by normal levels of ambient lighting should be avoided.

(3) In examinations resulting in images of high contrast (e.g., gastrointestinal studies) there may not always be a need for optimum image quality. Under such circumstances, in order to reduce patient dose, it may be desirable to have recourse to an alternative mode of operation using the automatic exposure rate control, whereby automatic variations in generator and tube output are biased in favour of changes in tube kilovoltage rather than tube current.

(4) Where image intensifier fluoroscopy incorporates a system of automatic exposure rate control, it is usual to have at least two settings of this control available. This permits X-ray examinations to be conducted (for the most part) at a low setting of the automatic control (e.g., giving 5–10 nC/kg per second at the intensifier input), and only when improved image quality is required would it be necessary to switch to the high setting (e.g., giving 26 nC/kg per second).

(5) Where fluoroscopic equipment incorporates an area exposure product meter, this provides a useful means of checking daily the consistency of radiation output of the X-ray tube and generator.

Table 4.   Parameters to be checked on fluoroscopic equipment

Recommended priority[a]	Text section No.	Item	Personnel category[b]	on installation	after repair	as necessary	A[c]	W[c]
				Testing required:				
A	5.4.1	Tube and generator	P/R	X	X	X	X	X
A	5.4.2	Automatic exposure rate control	P/R	X	X	X	X	X
A	5.4.3	Field size and distortion	P	X	X	X	X	
A	5.4.4	Beam collimation and alignment	P	X	X	X	X	
B	5.4.5	Conversion factor	P	X	X	X		
B	5.4.6	Contrast ratio veiling glare	P	X	X	X		
A	5.4.7	Grey scale test object	P	X	X	X	X	
A	5.4.8	Limiting resolution	P/R	X	X	X	X	X
A	5.4.9	Threshold contrast	P/R	X	X	X	X	X
A	5.4.10	Minimum visible detail versus contrast	P	X	X	X	X	

KEY: [a] A = essential; B = necessary for good practice.
      [b] P = physicist or engineer; R = radiographer or technician.
      [c] A = annually; W = weekly.

5.5 Special radiology equipment

Owing to special conditions of operation or use, a number of specific types of diagnostic radiological systems have been designated "special radiology equipment" in this guide. It is assumed that the general quality control techniques described in the previous sections of this chapter—covering the generator, X-ray tube with associated beam limiting device, image receptor and processing—will apply as appropriate. The items outlined in this section describe unique aspects of the special equipment that must be considered.

5.5.1 *Mammographic equipment: parameters to be checked* (Table 5)

Breast radiography presents a number of special considerations owing to the difficult task of visualizing objects of low radiographic contrast, in relation to surrounding tissue, and calcific bodies of small dimensions. This visualization task requires special consideration in the selection of X-ray tube type, tube potential, and filtration. A quality assurance programme for this type of equipment must deal with the operational factors that affect the spectra of the

Table 5. Parameters to be checked on mammographic equipment

Recom-mended priority[a]	Text para-graph No.	Item	Personnel category[b]	Testing required:					
				on instal-lation	after repair	as necess-ary	A[c]	M[c]	W[c]
A	(1)	Tube potential (kV$_p$)	P/R	X	X		X		
A	(1)	Half-value layer (HVL)	P/R	X	X		X		
A	(2)	Safelights	R	X	X	X			
A	(2)	Screens	R	X					X
A	(2)	Film/screen contact	R	X				X	
A	(3)	Plates (dark dusting)	R	X				X	

KEY: [a] A = essential.
  [b] P = physicist or engineer; R = radiographer or technician.
  [c] A = annually; M = monthly; W = weekly.

diagnostic beam. Special films, screens and cassettes, and/or electrostatic imaging systems are commonly used in mammography and require specific attention. Items of specific concern are outlined below.

(1) *Tube potential and filtration*

As with general radiographic equipment, tube potential (kVp) calibration and half-value layer (HVL) should be checked periodically (see Table 5). Checks of tube potential should focus on generator selections typically used in the clinic (25–35 kVp for film and 40–50 kVp for electrostatic image receptors). Half-value layer measurements should be made with the equipment configured as it is for mammography. For film, this may imply a molybdenum (Mo) filter in the beam on special-purpose mammographic units, or no added filtration on general radiographic systems used for mammography.

(2) *Film and screens*

For mammography, specially designed films, screens, and cassettes should be used. The quality assurance procedures for such systems include the use of proper safelights, routine cleaning of screens, checking for artefacts, and periodic testing for proper film/screen contact.

(3) *Electrostatic systems*

The quality assurance procedures for electrostatic imaging systems (i.e., xerography) include routine periodic dark dusting of the plates to check for powder deficiency spots and other artefacts, and periodic preventive maintenance checks of the processing system. Specific advice from the manufacturer with regard to proper set-up and operation should be obtained.

5.5.2 *Conventional tomography: parameters to be checked* (Table 6)

The mechanical complexity associated with conventional tomographic equipment requires special consideration in the establishment of a quality assurance programme. The following operational aspects of this type of equipment should be considered. General guidance regarding quality assurance for conventional tomographic equipment is given by Hendee & Rossi (*19*).

(1) *Verification of the accuracy of the tomographic cut level indicator*

Inaccuracy or nonreproducibility of the tomographic level or section indicator may result in deletion of information of diagnostic interest from the tomographic image.

(2) *Measurement of exposure angle (angle of swing)*

Inaccuracy or nonreproducibility of the tomographic exposure angle may result in tomographic sections that are too thick or too thin and will compromise the anticipated clinical goal.

(3) *Uniformity of radiation output*

Nonuniform exposure over the arc of motion of the tomographic unit yields an effective tomographic angle different from that indicated by the exposure angle indicator, together with an increased susceptibility of the tomographic unit to produce streaks in the image.

(4) *Tomographic movement configuration and mechanical stability*

For visualization of different anatomical features, tomographic sections of different thickness are employed. To facilitate this visualization, identical control settings on the tomographic unit should yield identical cut thicknesses.

Mechanical instability in the tomographic unit may result in tomographic images that do not reflect a flat section through the patient's anatomy. This loss of flatness may be interpreted incorrectly as an unusual anatomical configuration in the patient.

(5) *Resolution consistency*

The clarity of information in a tomographic image is critically dependent on the spatial resolution provided by the tomographic unit. Hence, tests should be performed periodically to ensure that no degradation of spatial resolution has occurred in the unit.

Table 6. Parameters to be checked on conventional tomographic equipment

Recommended priority[a]	Text paragraph No.	Item	Personnel category[b]	Testing required: on installation	after repair	S[c]
A	(1)	Cut level	P	X	X	X
A	(2)	Exposure angle	P	X	X	X
A	(3)	Exposure uniformity	P/R	X	X	X
A	(4)	Mechanical stability	P/R	X	X	X
A	(5)	Resolution	P/R	X	X	X

KEY: [a] A = essential.
[b] P = physicist or engineer; R = radiographer or technician.
[c] S = semi-annually.

5.5.3 Cineradiographic equipment: parameters to be checked (Table 7)

In general, quality assurance tests for fluoroscopy will apply for cineradiographic systems (1). The following additional items should be given specific consideration.

(1) *Beam restriction*
Special consideration should be given to ensuring that the X-ray beam is restricted to the useful area of the input phosphor. Significant overframing will increase patient dose and decrease image quality owing to higher levels of scattered radiation.

(2) *Alignment*
The cineradiographic field of view should be aligned with the visual field of the image intensifier and the potential of the recorded image field should be identified on the visual field of the image intensifier.

(3) *Resolution*
There should be periodic tests for overall system resolution.

(4) *Exposure rate at the input screen (surface) of the image intensifier*
Action should be taken if exposure rates are not of the order of 2–10 pC/kg per frame (26). Further reference to the manufacturer's instructions and input cine exposure set-up at installation should be made.

(5) *Automatic exposure control*
The system should be tested for reproducibility of performance.

(6) *Cleaning of optical components*
There should be periodic visual examination of the optical system. Manufacturers may recommend cleaning procedures which may require their assistance when major system disassembly is necessary. The high electrical potentials associated with the image tube may have an electrostatic precipitation effect causing an accelerated accumulation of dust in the optical system.

Table 7. Parameters to be checked on cineradiographic equipment

Recom-mended priority[a]	Text para-graph No.	Item	Personnel category[b]	Testing required:				
				on instal-lation	after repair	as necess-ary	A[c]	S[c]
A	(1)	Beam restriction	P	X	X	X		X
A	(2)	System alignment	P	X	X	X		X
A	(3)	System resolution	P	X	X	X		X
A	(4)	Exposure rate	P	X	X	X		X
A	(5)	Automatic expo-sure control	P	X	X	X		X
A	—	Camera/film	P/R	X	X	X		Every film change
A	(6)	Optical cleaning	P/R	X	X	X	X	
A	(7)	Camera shutter	P/R	X	X	X	X	

KEY: [a] A = essential.
      [b] P = physicist or engineer; R = radiographer or technician.
      [c] A = annually; S = semi-annually.

(7) *Camera shutter*

The camera shutter performance should be evaluated to ensure that it is functioning properly. Overexposure may result if the camera shutter is not appropriately synchronized with the X-ray pulse system.

5.5.4 *Computer tomography (CT) systems: parameters to be checked* (Table 8)

Computer tomography systems are complex devices involving many mechanical and electronic components that can affect image quality and equipment performance. Many of these items can often cause problems, but are difficult to test. It is therefore important to perform routine tests of overall imaging performance (*22*). Suboptimum results will reflect the existence of some problem in the imaging chain, which should be corrected by service personnel. Many of these tests can be performed using manufacturer-supplied phantoms.

(1) *Precision (noise)*

Precision, or noise, is defined as the variation of the CT number over an area of a uniform reference substance (usually water). It is measured by scanning a water-bath and measuring the standard deviation over an area of at least 1 cm^2 and dividing the result by the maximum CT number (usually 500 or 1000). The result should not be more than 0.5–1.0. Higher values may reflect poor detector performance, misalignment of X-ray beam and detector, insufficient X-ray output, or electrical noise.

Table 8. Parameters to be checked on computer tomography equipment

Recommended priority[a]	Text paragraph No.	Item	Personnel category[b]	Testing required: on installation	after repair	as necessary	A[c]	W[c]	D[c]
A	(1)	Precision	P/R	X	X	X			X
A	(2)	Uniformity	P/R	X	X	X			X
A	(3)	Accuracy/contrast	P/R	X	X	X	X		
A	(4)	Sensitivity	P	X	X	X	X		
A	(5)	Spatial resolution	P	X		X	X		
A	(6)	Artefacts	P/R	X		X			
B	(7)	Patient exposure	P	X		X		X	

KEY: [a] A = essential; B = necessary for good practice.
  [b] P = physicist or engineer; R = radiographer or technician.
  [c] A = annually; W = weekly; D = daily.

(2) *Uniformity*

Uniformity is defined as the consistency of the CT number for a uniform reference material (usually water) over the scan plane. It is determined by measuring the mean CT number of a scanned water-bath at several locations in the image and calculating the standard deviation. All measured points should fall within ± 2 standard deviations of the mean CT value. Failure of the system to meet this test could reflect beam-hardening artefacts.

(3) *Accuracy/contrast scale*

When a test object containing various materials (including water) is scanned at different times, the CT number for each material should not change and the CT number for water should be 0 ± 2.0. When these values change, improper X-ray generator calibration or other electronic problems may be indicated.

(4) *Sensitivity*

Sensitivity refers to the CT unit's capability to resolve objects of low subject contrast. Since sensitivity is CT's main strength, this is an especially important parameter. Sensitivity may be tested by using a phantom (several are commercially available) containing objects of various sizes and subject contrast and observing the smallest visible object of each contrast level. Usually an object of 1% subject contrast and 0.5–1.0 cm in size should be visible. Poor performance in this test is generally caused by the same factors that increase noise (see paragraph (1) above).

(5) *Spatial resolution*

Spatial resolution is most easily tested by scanning a "bar pattern" or "step pattern" test object and locating the smallest resolved spatial frequency. Acceptable performance depends on equipment type and can range from 2 to 3 line pairs per centimetre for some early generation scanners to over 10 pairs per centimetre for high-resolution scanners.

(6) *Artefacts*

Artefacts are defined as structures or features in an image that have usually been introduced by the equipment and are not present in the patient. This includes streaking, star patterns, and rings. Some artefacts, such as streaking and radiation stars, can be caused by sharp, high-contrast borders or metal in the patient. All others should be corrected by service personnel.

(7) *Patient exposure*

Image quality in CT is generally directly related to the amount of X-rays reaching the detectors and, therefore, to patient exposure. To avoid the pitfall of using high-dose scan settings to get the "prettiest" pictures, dose measurements for commonly used combinations of tube potential (kVp), current (mA), time, slice thickness, spacing, etc., should be made and the results posted.

5.5.5 *Dental equipment: parameters to be checked* (Table 9)

The majority of dental X-ray systems in current use are of relatively simple design. Dental equipment is singled out for consideration in this special equipment section because it is often operated by personnel who have only limited training in radiography. The nature of its design and use results in a low rate of replacement. Units of older design, often needing repair, are commonly found in clinical use. The following items are of key concern:

(1) *Stability of the tube head (consistent repositioning)*

Stabilizing the tube head to eliminate vibration and drifting prevents possible blurring and partial image formation in the finished radiograph.

(2) *Proper beam alignment*

Checking the alignment of the beam at the end of the position-indicating device (cone or cylinder) will help to minimize the chances of "cone cutting" in the finished radiograph.

Table 9.   Parameters to be checked on dental X-ray equipment

Recom-mended priority[a]	Text para-graph No.	Item	Personnel category[b]	on instal-lation	after repair	as necess-ary	A[c]	S[c]	M[c]
A	(1)	Tube head stability	R	X	X	X			X
A	(2)	Beam alignment	R	X	X	X	X		
A	(3)	Technique factor	P	X	X	X	X		
A	(4)	Exposure reproduci-bility	P	X	X	X	X		
A	(5)	HVL	P	X	X	X	X		
A	(6)	ESE	P R	X	X	X		X	X

KEY: [a] A = essential.
    [b] P = physicist or engineer; R = radiographer or technician.
    [c] A = annually; S = semi-annually; M = monthly.

(3) *Technique factor accuracy*

The absolute accuracy of the operational technique factors—tube potential (kVp), current (mA), and time—are less important in dental than in medical radiology. Where checks reveal a major variation ($+10\%$) this should be corrected by the equipment service engineer.

(4) *Exposure reproducibility*

Variations in output under the operational conditions used in clinical applications should be checked. Units consistent with modern design can be expected to have a coefficient of variation of not more than 0.05. (The coefficient of variation is usually based on measurements from a series of 10 exposures and estimated using the following equation:

$$C = \frac{s}{\overline{X}} = \frac{1}{\overline{X}} \left[\sum_{i=1}^{n} \frac{(X_i - X)^2}{n-1} \right]^{\frac{1}{2}}$$

where s = estimated standard deviation of the population, $\overline{X}$ = mean value of observations in sample, X_i = ith observation sampled, and n = number of observations sampled.) If variations greater than this are obtained, further investigation should be undertaken to identify the cause, which may be related to variations in the tube potential, current, and/or exposure time.

(5) *Half-value layer (HVL)—beam quality*

Evaluating the beam quality by means of half-value layer measurements will determine the total filtration (inherent and added). HVL measurements are useful in detecting X-ray tube deterioration.

(6) *Machine output (patient entrance skin exposure—ESE)*

A comparison of cone tip exposures to a predetermined range of acceptable exposures will assist in the selection of appropriate exposure factors needed to produce radiographs of optimum density and contrast, when recommended film processing procedures are followed. In some countries scientific/professional societies or governmental agencies have provided assistance in this area. If such assistance is not available, the aid of an X-ray engineer/physicist should be sought (*14*).

5.6 Photofluorographic equipment

Photofluorographic X-ray units are still in use in many parts of the world. Their primary applications have been for mass screening for the detection of chest diseases, including primary tuberculosis, pneumoconiosis, and silicosis. Patient exposure from these units is significantly greater than from conventional film/screen radiography. Caution must be taken to assure that units of this type are operated at the minimum exposure levels consistent with the acquisition of adequate diagnostic information.

5.6.1 *Unit design*

Systems with mirror optics or fast lens systems have been shown to be capable of operating in the range of 25–50 mC/kg per chest. Consideration should be given to the appropriate selection of fast film, the proper grid, and operational X-ray technique factors, so that, for patients of average dimensions, exposures in this range are obtained.

5.6.2 *Periodic checks*

Units should be checked on a regular basis to verify proper operational conditions. An exposure with a phantom should be made to check patient exposure levels. Attention should be given to items that may cause a decrease in system performance. The condition of the screen (phosphor) and dirt on the optical system are important items to consider.

6. Training requirements

QUALITY assurance procedures in diagnostic radiology have been developed in the last few years and are not at present taught on a routine basis to persons working in this field, such as radiologists, radiographers, medical physicists, and X-ray engineers. It is therefore essential that training programmes for the introduction and wide application of quality assurance procedures in diagnostic radiology should be established for the various categories of personnel in need of such training.

However, the groups of people concerned should be encouraged to make the maximum use of elements relating to quality assurance in their basic professional training, and such professional training should, in future, incorporate something of the basic concepts inherent in quality assurance programmes.

6.1 Categories of personnel and training

In view of the variety of backgrounds and responsibilities of the categories of personnel to be trained in quality assurance procedures, training should be provided for the following groups:

(1) radiographers or medical radiology technicians, who have to perform on a routine basis the techniques recommended throughout this report;

(2) radiologists;

(3) other medical personnel who perform radiodiagnostic procedures on a more or less routine basis—dentists, physiologists, gastroenterologists, orthopaedists, chiropractors, etc.; and

(4) medical and health physicists, X-ray engineers, and engineering technicians.

Although the training requirements of each group will differ, the relevant training curricula will contain some common fundamentals.

6.2 Practical versus theoretical training

In general, all training in quality assurance procedures should be practically oriented, with a minimum of formal teaching. Formal teaching should be restricted to that necessary to achieve an understanding of the physical and physicochemical parameters investigated, and the maximum amount of time should be devoted to the direct application of the procedures and an evaluation of results. Using this approach, the training could be brief, but at the same time the number of trainees on each course should be restricted in accordance with the facilities available.

6.3 Special versus integrated training

In the case of personnel already in posts with basic levels of training that did not include quality assurance, there is a need to establish special courses for quality assurance procedures.

At the same time it would be valuable to review the present curricula of all schools or other institutions where medical radiology technicians, radiologists, medical and health physicists, X-ray engineers, and engineering technicians are trained and to include the teaching of quality assurance in those curricula. Such an integrated training would produce future specialists who are capable and aware of the importance of performing quality assurance procedures, and would gradually reduce the need for special courses to teach new techniques or for refresher training schemes.

6.4 Suggestions for curricula for different types of training

As mentioned in section 6.1, the different types of courses will be designed for various categories of personnel with particular tasks in the quality assurance programme and with a background which is specific to each category. Some suggestions concerning the adaptation necessary for such curricula are given below.

6.4.1 *Training for medical radiology technicians*

Medical radiology technicians will have to play a key role in the basic (routine) quality assurance procedures in radiography (see sections 5.2 and 5.3). A full understanding of the procedures and parameters relevant to the performance of imaging systems should be included in the curricula for this category. Emphasis has to be placed on all aspects dealing with the most common procedures in quality assurance and on the full understanding of factors, including patient exposures, that lead to unacceptable results and ways of correction.

6.4.2 *Training for radiologists*

As a user of the diagnostic image, the radiologist must be aware of all essential factors that influence the image quality and patient exposure and induce artefacts, etc. He has to know the quality assurance procedures in principle, but emphasis should be on the parameters that can objectively describe the diagnostic quality of the image and on causes that could explain failures in obtaining an image of acceptable diagnostic quality. Additional knowledge and internationally accepted data are needed for an adequate definition of the "diagnostic quality of images" (see Chapter 3).

6.4.3 Training for other medical personnel using radiological techniques

These should have a curriculum with a content which is balanced between that of the courses outlined in sections 6.4.1 and 6.4.2, depending on their particular need.

6.4.4 Training for medical and health physicists, X-ray engineers and engineering technicians

This group would need the most complex training, producing specialists in quality assurance procedures who are able to carry out a wide range of techniques, assess performance of imaging systems, and (where appropriate) repair the faulty parts of the equipment.

It will be necessary for these specialists to collaborate with all the other categories of staff specified above, in order that they may play a major role in the training of all personnel in quality assurance procedures.

6.4.5 Teaching methods and manuals

Methods of teaching must be flexible and accommodate such factors as variations in the background knowledge of trainees and local facilities. The curriculum must include practical demonstrations of quality assurance procedures.

The effectiveness of the training should be assessed. Possible methods include comparison of image quality, regular reject (retake) analysis, and comparisons of dose levels for imaging.

Instruction manuals and teaching aids should be an integral part of the training programme. The production and regular updating of these manuals should be encouraged.

Comparative studies of X-ray image quality on a local, regional, or international basis are important and should have an impact on the aims of training and the motivation for developing and maintaining programmes.

6.5 National versus international training

The variety and high degree of specialization implied by training in quality assurance raise the problem that this will not always be possible within the country. It is desirable that basic-level training of medical radiology technicians and other persons involved in quality assurance procedures should be organized nationally. In countries in which radiologists are locally trained, the courses outlined in sections 6.4.1 and 6.4.2 could be arranged. In countries in which this is not the case, the national authority in charge of quality assurance in diagnostic radiology (e.g., the national radiation protection service) could arrange such courses, using a specialist trained abroad.

The training of medical and health physicists, X-ray engineers, and engineering technicians could be conducted in countries in which adequate technical knowledge and suitable facilities exist. In the absence of these resources, such training would have to be organized on an international basis. Efforts should be made to identify the places where courses could be held, to draw up appropriate curricula and training programmes, to arrange the courses, and to encourage countries to send their personnel for training. On their return home, these specialists would be the initiators of quality assurance programmes in their own countries and could also train local staff.

7. Recapitulation

DIAGNOSTIC radiology provides a valuable input into health care delivery. Effective use of this technology can only be assured through a planned and systematic approach. Quality assurance procedures dealing with equipment performance are a key element in this systematic approach.

The following sections draw attention to features considered to be of special importance to all those concerned in implementing quality assurance programmes—the staff of diagnostic radiological facilities, manufacturers, professional/scientific societies, national authorities, and international bodies.

7.1 Radiological facilities

The quality assurance programme of a diagnostic radiological facility should contain the elements listed in sections 7.1.1–7.1.10. The extent to which each element of the quality assurance programme is implemented should be determined on the basis of an analysis of the facility's objectives and resources, conducted by qualified personnel. The analysis should be designed to show whether the expected benefits in improved image quality, radiation exposure reduction, and/or financial savings will compensate for the resources required to implement the programme.

7.1.1 Responsibility

(1) The owner or practitioner in charge of the facility has primary responsibility for implementing and maintaining the quality assurance programme.

(2) Generally, staff technologists (medical radiology technicians or other X-ray equipment operators) should be assigned a basic quality assurance role by the practitioner in charge—for example, responsibility for specific quality control monitoring and maintenance techniques, or quality administration procedures—provided that they have had the requisite training or experience. The staff technologists should also be responsible for identifying problems or potential problems requiring actions beyond their scope and reporting such

problems to the practitioner in charge, or his or her representative, who should then resolve the difficulties with intra- or extramural assistance.

(3) When available, physicists, X-ray engineers, supervisory technologists, or other personnel with technical supervisory responsibilities should have a major role in the quality assurance programme. These specialized personnel may be assigned responsibility for day-to-day administration of the programme, carry out monitoring duties beyond the level of training of the staff technologist, or—if desired by the facility—relieve the staff technologists of some or all of their basic monitoring duties. Staff service engineers may also be assigned responsibility for certain preventive or corrective maintenance actions.

(4) Responsibility for certain quality control techniques and corrective measures may be assigned to qualified personnel from outside the facility, such as consultants or industrial representatives, provided there is a written agreement clearly specifying these services.

(5) In large facilities, responsibility for long-range planning of quality assurance goals and activities should be assigned to a quality assurance committee as described in section 7.1.9.

(6) Responsibility and authority for the overall quality assurance programme, as well as for monitoring, evaluation, and corrective measures, should be specified and recorded in a quality assurance manual.

7.1.2 Purchase specifications

Before purchasing new equipment, the staff of the diagnostic radiological facility should determine the desired performance specifications for the equipment. Initially these specifications may be stated in terms of the desired performance of the equipment, or prospective vendors may simply be asked to provide the performance specifications of items from their equipment line that can perform the desired functions. In either case, the responses of the prospective vendors should serve as the basis for negotiations to establish the final purchase specifications, taking into account the state of the art and balancing the need for the specified performance levels with the cost of the equipment to meet them. The final purchase specifications should be in writing and should include performance specifications. The availability of experienced service personnel should also be taken into consideration in making the final purchase decisions, and any servicing agreements should be incorporated into the written purchase specifications. After the equipment is installed, the facility should conduct a testing programme, as defined in its purchase specifications, to ensure that the equipment meets the agreed specifications, including the relevant regulatory requirements. The purchase specifications and the records of the acceptance testing should be retained throughout the life of the equipment for comparison with later results, in order to assess the continued acceptability of the equipment's performance.

7.1.3 Monitoring and maintenance

A routine quality control monitoring and maintenance system incorporating state-of-the-art procedures should be established and conducted on a regular schedule. Monitoring permits the evaluation of the performance of the facility's X-ray system(s) in terms of the standards for image quality established by the facility (as described in section 7.1.4) and compliance with applicable regulatory requirements. The maintenance programme should include corrective maintenance and preventive maintenance.

(1) The parameters to be monitored in a facility should be determined by each individual facility on the basis of an analysis of expected benefits and cost. Such factors as the size and resources of the facility, the type of examinations conducted, and the quality assurance problems that have already occurred in that facility or in similar establishments should be taken into account in setting up the monitoring system. The monitoring frequency should also be based on need and will vary for different parameters.

(2) Although the parameters to be monitored will change from facility to facility, every diagnostic radiological facility should consider monitoring the following five key components of the radiological system:

(a) performance characteristics of the X-ray generator;

(b) beam limiting device;

(c) image receptor (films, cassettes and screens, image intensifier, etc.) and grids;

(d) darkroom and processing; and

(e) viewing equipment.

Guidance with respect to the specific elements that should be accorded a high priority for inclusion in a facility programme and their suggested frequency of monitoring are given in Chapter 5.

(3) The maintenance programme should include both preventive and corrective aspects.

(a) *Preventive maintenance.* Preventive maintenance should be performed on a regular basis, with the goal of preventing breakdowns due to defects not detectable by routine monitoring.

(b) *Corrective maintenance.* For maximum effectiveness, the quality assurance programme should make provision (see section 7.1.5) for detecting the development of actual or potential problems, which corrective maintenance can then eliminate before they have any major impact on patient care.

7.1.4 *Criteria for image quality*

Criteria for acceptable image quality should be established. Ideally these should be objective (for example, acceptability limits for the variations of parameter values); but they may be subjective (for example, the opinions of professional personnel in cases where adequate objective standards cannot or have not as yet been defined—see Chapter 3). These standards should be routinely reviewed and redefined as necessary (see section 7.1.10).

Although detailed numerical criteria for defining image quality are difficult to establish, some effort should be made to do so. For example, methods that will allow scientific study of the subject and will yield results in a form that is understandable and useful to the clinical community should be investigated (see section 7.5.4, for activities at the international level).

7.1.5 Evaluation

The facility's quality assurance programme should include the means for two stages of evaluation.

(1) At the first stage, the results of the monitoring procedures should be used to evaluate the performance of the radiological system(s), in order to determine whether corrective actions are needed to ensure that the image quality consistently meets the established criteria. This evaluation should include analysis of trends in the monitoring data as well as the use of the data on a day-to-day basis. Monitoring data should also be compared with the purchase specifications and acceptance testing results for the equipment in question.

(2) At the second stage, the facility's quality assurance programme should include means for evaluating the effectiveness of the programme itself, such as ongoing studies of the retake rate and the causes of retakes, examination of equipment repair and replacement costs, subjective evaluation of the radiographs being produced, occurrence of and reasons for complaints by radiologists and an analysis of trends in the results of monitoring procedures (e.g., sensitometric studies).

7.1.6 Records

The programme should include provisions for keeping records of the results of the monitoring techniques, any variations detected, the corrective measures applied, and the effectiveness of these measures. The facility should view these records as a tool for maintaining an effective quality assurance programme; they should also be made available to vendors to help them to provide better service. More importantly, the data should be the basis for the evaluation and the reviews suggested in sections 7.1.5 and 7.1.10.

7.1.7 Written facility procedures

A written protocol describing the facility's quality assurance programme should be developed in a format permitting convenient revision as needed, and should be made readily available to all personnel. The content of the protocol should be determined by the staff of the facility, but the following items are thought to be essential:

(1) A list of the individuals responsible for monitoring and maintenance techniques.

(2) A list of the parameters to be monitored and the frequency of monitoring.

(3) A description of the standards, quality criteria, or limits of acceptability which have been established for each monitored parameter.

(4) A brief description of the procedures to be used for monitoring each parameter.

(5) A description of the procedures to be followed when difficulties requiring correction are detected.

(6) A list of the publications in which detailed instructions for monitoring and maintenance procedures can be found. Copies of these publications should be readily available to the entire staff, but they should be separate from the manual.

(7) A list of the records, with sample forms, that the facility staff has decided should be kept. The staff should also determine and note in the manual the length of time each type of record should be kept before being discarded.

7.1.8 *Training*

The programme should include appropriate training for all personnel—radiographers, physicists/engineers, and physicians—with quality assurance responsibilities (see Chapter 6). This should comprise both training before the quality assurance responsibilities are assumed and continuing education to keep the personnel concerned up to date. Special consideration should be given to the availability of appropriate training aids—manuals, reports, courses, etc. Efforts may be required at the facility level if appropriate training materials are not available from manufacturers, scientific/professional societies, national groups, or international bodies.

7.1.9 *Quality assurance committee*

In a large facility where it would be impracticable for all staff members to meet for planning purposes, the establishment of a quality assurance committee should be considered. The committee's primary function would be to maintain lines of communication among all groups with quality assurance and/or image production or interpretation responsibilities. For maximum communication, all departments with X-ray equipment should be represented. The committee may also have policy-making duties, such as assigning quality assurance responsibilities, maintaining acceptable standards of quality, and periodically reviewing programme effectiveness. Alternatively, the duties of this committee could be delegated to an already existing committee, such as the radiation safety committee. In smaller facilities, all staff members should participate in the committee's tasks. The quality assurance committee should report directly to the head of the radiology department, or, in facilities where more than one department operates X-ray equipment, to the chief medical officer of the facility. The committee should meet on a regular basis.

7.1.10 *Review*

The facility's quality assurance programme should be reviewed by the quality assurance committee and/or the practitioner in charge to determine whether its effectiveness could be improved. Items suggested for inclusion in the review are:

(1) The reports of the monitoring and maintenance techniques, to ensure that these are being performed effectively and on schedule. These reports should be reviewed at least quarterly.

(2) The monitoring and maintenance techniques and their schedules, to ensure that they continue to be appropriate and in step with the latest developments in quality assurance. They should be updated at least annually.

(3) The standards for image quality, to ensure that they are consistent with the state of the art and the needs and resources of the facility. These standards should be reviewed at least annually.

(4) The results of the evaluations of the effectiveness of the quality assurance procedures, to determine whether changes need to be made. This determination should be made at least annually.

(5) The quality assurance protocols, to determine whether revision is needed. The protocols should be reviewed at least annually.

(6) Intercomparison of the approach and effectiveness of quality assurance programmes by outside groups (scientific/professional societies, national authorities, or international bodies), to identify areas where improvements can be made at the facility level.

7.2 Manufacturers

The expertise of the manufacturer regarding the design and operation of the radiology equipment should be made available, so that appropriate testing programmes can be developed and implemented. The manufacturer's service representatives may provide valuable assistance to clinical facilities that do not have adequate technical staff to plan and implement an effective quality assurance programme.

7.2.1 *Specific test protocols*

Manufacturers should provide information on the specific design or operational characteristics of their equipment so that appropriate testing programmes can be developed.

7.2.2 *Special radiology equipment*

For special radiology equipment, such as computer tomographic units, the manufacturers should develop appropriate quality assurance procedures and provide instructions for their use.

7.3 Scientific/professional societies

Scientific/professional bodies should work through their membership to provide information and assistance regarding quality assurance. Effective interchange between groups (technologists, physicists/engineers, physicians, manufacturers, and governmental authorities) can be facilitated through coordination of efforts by representatives of the individual groups.

7.3.1 *Availability of information*

Through the convening of meetings and the publishing of scientific papers and manuals, etc., information on quality assurance can be made available to facility personnel. Information provided by a scientific/professional society is often more positively received by its members than that provided through other sources.

7.3.2 *Training*

Specific emphasis should be placed on providing appropriate training materials and a reference manual. Scientific/professional societies should emphasize the need for, and facilitate the availability of, appropriate training. Participation by members can be encouraged through the inclusion of an accredited or certificated quality assurance examination, and through official recognition of further participation, where applicable.

7.3.3 *Special guidance*

Specialized fields—for example, dentistry, chiropractic, and paediatrics—in which only a limited part of the body is X-rayed, or in which equipment of a specific type is employed, should develop guidance appropriate to their specific practices and technical resources.

7.4 National authorities

Radiological authorities at the national level can provide valuable assistance to the clinical community. Governmental authorities can effectively supplement their usual basic regulatory conditions regarding design, installation, and radiation safety with nonregulatory guidance in quality assurance (*39*).

7.4.1 *Area-specific guidance*

Since the type of equipment and the level of knowledge are known to vary in different parts of the world, the national authority can provide valuable assistance in giving appropriate guidance to clinical users in their region.

7.4.2 *Training*

In many cases, input at the national level will assure that appropriate training is available. This may be provided directly or through the encouragement of scientific/professional groups and manufacturers.

7.4.3 *Monitoring*

The national authorities are in a unique position to review the status of quality assurance programmes on a facility-to-facility basis. Monitoring programmes that look at the practices in a large cross-section of a country's radiological facilities can provide valuable information regarding areas where additional emphasis should be placed.

7.4.4 Coordination

Quality assurance programmes require the participation of a number of different classifications of personnel and groups. Efforts at the national level can assist the different interest groups in integrating their various efforts.

7.5 International participation

The 1980 Workshop demonstrated the wide interest in quality assurance programmes for diagnostic radiology. Various international, governmental and nongovernmental organizations were involved, including the World Health Organization, the Commission of the European Communities, the Federal Health Office of the Federal Republic of Germany, the International Electrotechnical Commission; the International Society of Radiographers and Radiological Technicians, and the International Society of Radiology. It is expected that this interest will gradually increase and that WHO will act as a focal point for mobilizing the necessary scientific action and resources to promote activities involving the international and national bodies concerned. A number of areas where international efforts would be effective have been identified.

7.5.1 Intercomparison of quality assurance at the international level

The collection and publication of comparative information on quality assurance activities at the national level should be considered, and the results of efforts to reduce the number of ineffectual procedures and improve diagnostic quality should be studied.

7.5.2 International recommendations

Recommendations for quality protocols, techniques, and procedures as a technical basis for quality assurance programmes to be applied at the national level should be developed. Activities at the international level facilitate the collection and distribution of appropriate information.

7.5.3 Training

Specific emphasis should be placed on training. This training effort might include the organization of seminars, workshops, and training courses at the regional or global level.

7.5.4 Standardization of image quality

Attempts should be made to establish internationally accepted guidelines/criteria for image quality (see section 7.1.4).

REFERENCES

1. ADDISON, S. J. ET AL. Diagnostic X-ray survey procedures for fluoroscopic installations—III: Cinefluorographic units. *Health physics*, **35**: 845 (1978).
2. ARAUJO, A. M. C. ET AL. Diagnostic X-ray equipment evaluation in Brazil. *XIV Congresso Internacional de Radiologia. Resumos.* Rio de Janeiro, 1977, p. 602.
3. ARDRAN, G. M. & CROOKS, H. E. Checking diagnostic X-ray beam quality. *British journal of radiology*, **41**: 193 (1968).
4. ARDRAN, G. M. ET AL. Testing X-ray cassettes for film intensifying screen contact. *Radiography*, **35**: 143 (1969).
5. BEIDEMAN, R. W. ET AL. A study to develop a rating system and evaluate dental radiographs submitted to a third party carrier. *Journal of the American Dental Association*, **93**: 1010 (1976).
6. BERRY, R. J. & OLIVER, R. Spoilt films in X-ray departments and radiation exposure to the public from medical radiology. *British journal of radiology*, **49**: 475 (1977).
7. BROWN, M. R. Preventative maintenance reduces X-ray equipment costs. *Dimensions in the health service*, **51**: 3 (1974).
8. BULLEN, M. A. & BYE, R. T. Raycheck—a new radiological test instrument for quality assurance. *Radiography*, **45**: 278 (1979).
9. BUNGE, R. E. ET AL. The need for quality assurance in diagnostic radiology. Abstract presented at the *Ninth Annual Midyear Topical Symposium of the Health Physics Society, 9–12 February, 1976*, Boulder, Colorado. *Health Physics*, **31**(6): 565, 1976.
10. BURKHART, R. L. *Quality assurance programs for diagnostic radiology facilities.* Washington, DC, United States Food and Drug Administration, 1980 (DHEW Publication—FDA 80-8110).
11. COHEN, G. ET AL. The effects of the film/screen combination on tomographic image quality. *Radiology*, **129**: 515 (1978).
12. GILLAN, G. D. ET AL. The use of an anthropomorphic chest phantom. In: *Optimization of chest radiology*. Washington, DC, United States Food and Drug Administration, 1980 (DHHS publication 80-8124).
13. GOLDMAN, L. W. & BEECH, S. *Analysis of retakes: Understanding, managing, and using an analysis of retakes program for quality assurance.* Washington, DC, United States Food and Drug Administration, 1979 (DHEW Publication—FDA 79-8097).
14. GRATT, B. M. Xeroradiography of dental structures. III—Pilot clinical studies. *Oral surgery, oral medicine, and oral pathology*, **48**: 276 (1979).
15. GREENING, J. R. Testing X-ray equipment by examining emitted X-rays. *Radiography*, **25**: 199 (1959).
16. HALL, C. L. Economic analysis of a quality control program. Application of optical instrumentation in medicine, VI. *Proceedings of the Society of Photo-optical Instrumentation Engineers*, **127**: 271 (1977).
17. HENDEE, W. R. & ROSSI, R. P. *Quality assurance for radiographic X-ray units and associated equipment.* Washington, DC, United States Food and Drug Administration, 1979 (DHEW Publication—FDA 79-8094).
18. HENDEE, W. R. & ROSSI, R. P. *Quality assurance for fluoroscopic X-ray units and associated equipment.* Washington, DC, United States Food and Drug Administration, 1980 (DHEW Publication—FDA 80-8095).

19. HENDEE, W. R. & ROSSI, R. P. *Quality assurance for conventional tomographic X-ray units.* Washington, DC, United States Food and Drug Administration, 1980 (DHEW Publication—FDA 80-8096).
20. HOSPITAL PHYSICISTS' ASSOCIATION. *Measurement of the performance characteristics of diagnostic X-ray systems used in medicine. Part I—X-ray tubes and generators.* London, 1980 (Topic Group Report, No. 32).
21. HOSPITAL PHYSICISTS' ASSOCIATION [*Idem*] *Part II—X-ray image intensifier television systems.* London, 1981 (Topic Group Report, No. 32).
22. HOSPITAL PHYSICISTS' ASSOCIATION. [*Idem*] *Part III—Computed tomography X-ray scanners.* London, 1981 (Topic Group Report, No. 32).
23. HOSPITAL PHYSICISTS' ASSOCIATION. [*Idem*] *Part IV—Film, screens and autoprocessors,* London (in press) (Topic Group Report, No. 32).
24. HOSPITAL PHYSICISTS' ASSOCIATION. *The physics of radiodiagnosis.* London, 1976 (Scientific Report Series, No. 6).
25. INTERNATIONAL COMMISSION ON RADIOLOGICAL PROTECTION. *Protection of the patient in X-ray diagnosis.* Oxford, Pergamon Press (in press) (Publication No. 16, revised).
26. INTERNATIONAL COMMISSION ON RADIATION UNITS AND MEASUREMENTS. *Cameras for image intensifier fluorography.* Washington, DC, 1969 (Report No. 15).
27. INTERNATIONAL ELECTROTECHNICAL COMMISSION. *Entrance field size of electro-optical image intensifiers.* Geneva, 1975 (Publication No. 520).
28. INTERNATIONAL ELECTROTECHNICAL COMMISSION. *Determination of luminance distribution of electro-optical image intensifiers.* Geneva, 1977 (Publication No. 572).
29. INTERNATIONAL ELECTROTECHNICAL COMMISSION. *Measurement of conversion factor of electro-optical image intensifiers.* Geneva, 1977 (Publication No. 573).
30. INTERNATIONAL ELECTROTECHNICAL COMMISSION. *Area exposure product meter.* Geneva, 1977 (Publication No. 580).
31. INTERNATIONAL ELECTROTECHNICAL COMMISSION. *Determination of the image disrotation of electro-optical X-ray image intensifiers.* Geneva, 1981 (Publication No. 62B-66).
32. JACOBSON, A. F. ET AL. Test cassette for measuring peak tube potential of diagnostic X-ray machines. *Medical physics*, 3: 19 (1976).
33. MCKINLAY, A. & MCCAULEY, B. Spoilt films in X-ray departments. *British journal of radiology*, 50: 233–234 (1977).
34. METZ, C. E. Basic principles of ROC analysis. *Seminars in nuclear medicine.* New York, Grune & Stratton, 1978, Vol. 8, No. 4, pp. 283–289.
35. METZ, C. E. Applications of ROC analysis in diagnostic image evaluation. In: Haus, A. G. ed. *The physics of medical imaging: Recording system, measurements and techniques.* New York, American Institute of Physics, 1979.
36. MIDWEST REGIONAL EDUCATION COMMITTEE OF THE AMERICAN HOSPITAL RADIOLOGY ADMINISTRATORS. *Equipment specifications and performance standards.* (Available from: Wheeler, W. W., Grant Hospital, 550 W. Webster, Chicago, IL 60614, USA.)
37. MORGAN, R. H. & GEHRET, E. F., JR. *Gonad exposure in medical radiography: A handbook of scatter/primary exposure ratios.* Rockville, MD, United States Public Health Service, 1971 (BRH/DMRE Contract Report: DHEW—PH 86-68-63).
38. NATIONAL COUNCIL ON RADIATION PROTECTION AND MEASUREMENTS. *Medical X-ray and gamma-ray protection for energies up to 10 MeV—Equipment design and use.* Washington, DC, 1968 (NCRP Report No. 33).

39. NORWEGIAN SOCIETY OF MEDICAL RADIATION PHYSICS. *Quality assurance control for X-ray diagnostic equipment. (A catalogue of recommended methods and necessary measuring equipment).* Østeraas, State Institute of Radiation Hygiene, 1980.
40. PROTO, A. V. & LANE, E. J. 350 kVp Chest radiographs: Review and comparison with 120 kVp. *American journal of roentgenology,* **130**: 859 (1978).
41. SHOWALTER, C. K. ET AL. An analysis of film/screen combinations and patient exposures from nationwide evaluation of X-ray trends (NEXT). Application of optical instrumentation in medicine, VI. *Proceedings of the Society of Photo-optical Instrumentation Engineers,* **127**: 126 (1977).
42. SICKLES, E. A. ET AL. Comparison of laboratory and clinical evaluation of mammographic screen–film systems. Application of optical instrumentation in medicine, VI. *Proceedings of the Society of Photo-optical Instrumentation Engineers,* **127**: 30 (1977).
43. STARCHMAN, D. E. ET AL. The role of kVp accuracy of diagnostic X-ray units and other performance parameters in quality assurance. Application of optical instrumentation in medicine, V. *Proceedings of the Society of Photo-optical Instrumentation Engineers,* **96**: 31 (1976).
44. STARCHMAN, D. E. ET AL. Linearity of exposure with indicated time and current for diagnostic radiology units. *Radiology,* **122**: 489 (1977).
45. STEINER, R. M. ET AL. A comparative analysis of 350 kVp and 120 kVp chest radiography. In: *Optimization of chest radiography.* Washington, DC, United States Food and Drug Administration, 1980 (DHHS Publication—FDA 80-8124).
46. SWETS, J. A. ROC analysis applied to the evaluation of medical imaging techniques. *Investigative radiology,* **41** (20): 109 (1979).
47. SWETS, J. A. & PICKET, R. M. *Evaluation of diagnostic devices in clinical medicine: A general protocol.* Cambridge, MA, Bolt, Beranek & Newman, 1979 (Report No. 3819).
48. THORNBY, J. R. ET AL. A methodology for comparison of quality of radiological images from different screen/film combinations based on radiologists' subjective judgements. Application of optical instrumentation in medicine, VI. *Proceedings of the Society of Photo-optical Instrumentation Engineers,* **127**: 24 (1977).
49. TROUT, E. D. ET AL. Analysis of the rejection rate of chest radiographs obtained during the coal mine black lung program. *Radiology,* **109**: 25 (1973).
50. VUCICH, J. J. The role of anatomic criteria in the evaluation of radiographic images. In: Haus, A. G. ed., *The physics of medical imaging: Recording system measurements and techniques.* New York, American Institute of Physics, 1979.
51. VUCICH, J. J. ET AL. Use of anatomical criteria in screen/film selection for portable chest X-ray procedures. In: *Optimization of chest radiography.* Washington, DC, United States Food and Drug Administration, 1980 (DHSS—FDA 80-8124).
52. WHITTAKER, L. R. *Quality control in X-ray departments at Kenyan district hospitals.* Unpublished report to WHO, 1980. (Available from: Radiation Medicine, World Health Organization, 1211 Geneva 27, Switzerland).

Annex 1

Definitions of terms

The definitions of terms given below apply to the terms as used in this guide, and are not necessarily valid for other purposes.

Acceptance inspection (acceptance test)
Inspection to determine whether an item delivered or offered for delivery is acceptable (ISO 3534-1977). Such inspection may include tests carried out following the installation of equipment to determine whether it has been manufactured and installed in accordance with the agreed technical specifications; the results of these tests provide reference values against which the future performance of the equipment may be assessed when routine testing is undertaken.

Diagnostic radiological facility
Any establishment in which an X-ray system is used in any procedure that includes irradiation of any part of the human body for the purpose of diagnosis or visualization. This includes a wide range of facilities, from dental units to hospital departments of radiology.

Quality administration procedures
Managerial procedures for ensuring that monitoring techniques are properly performed and evaluated and that appropriate corrective measures are taken when the results show them to be necessary. These procedures provide the organizational framework for the quality assurance programme.

Quality assurance
All those planned and systematic actions necessary to provide adequate confidence that a structure, system or component will perform satisfactorily in service (ISO 6215-1980). Satisfactory performance in service implies the optimum quality of the entire diagnostic process—i.e., the consistent production of adequate diagnostic information with minimum exposure of both patients and personnel.

Quality assurance programme
The overall management and procedures covering the quality assurance actions for the execution of a specific contract or project (ISO 6215-1980). It is an organized activity designed to provide quality assurance in diagnostic radiology, and includes both quality control techniques and quality administration procedures. The nature and extent of this activity will vary with the size and type of the facility, the types of examination conducted, and other factors.

Quality control
The set of operations (programming, coordinating, carrying out) intended
to maintain or to improve quality [. . .] (ISO 3534-1977). As applied to a
diagnostic procedure, it covers monitoring, evaluation, and maintenance at
optimum levels of all characteristics of performance that can be defined,
measured, and controlled.

References

International Organization for Standardization. *Statistics—vocabulary and symbols*,
    Geneva, 1977 (International Standard ISO 3534-1977).
International Organization for Standardization. *Nuclear power plants—quality
    assurance*, Geneva, 1980 (International Standard ISO 6215-1980).

Annex 2

Participants in the Neuherberg Workshop

Dr L. K. Anderson, X-ray Department, National Institute of Radiation Protection, Stockholm, Sweden

Dr G. M. Ardran, University Department of Radiology, Radcliffe Infirmary, Oxford, England

Dr A. Bäumel, Institute for Radiation Hygiene, Federal Health Office, Neuherberg, Federal Republic of Germany

Dr J. Brederhoff, Radiation Medicine, WHO, Geneva Switzerland

Mr J. A. Den Boer, Hamburg, Federal Republic of Germany (*representing the International Electrotechnical Commission*)

Dr G. Drexler, Society for Radiation and Environmental Research, Neuherberg, Federal Republic of Germany

Dr H. Eriskat, Commission of the European Communities, Plateau du Kirchberg, Luxembourg

Dr J. Flatby, State Institute of Radiation Hygiene, Østeraas, Norway

Miss M. Frank, London, England (*representing the International Society of Radiographers and Radiological Technicians*)

Professor G. Hagemann, Institute of Clinical Radiology, Section of Experimental Radiology, Hanover Medical School, Hanover, Federal Republic of Germany

Dr E. T. Henshaw, Regional Radiation Protection Service, Mersey Regional Health Authority, Liverpool, England

Dr O. Hjardemaal, National Institute of Radiation Hygiene, Copenhagen, Denmark

Dr H. W. Julius, Organization for Applied Scientific Research, Arnheim, Netherlands

Professor F. Kossel, Institute for Radiation Hygiene, Federal Health Office, Neuherberg, Federal Republic of Germany

Dr G. Lang, CHF Müller, Medico-Technical Systems, Branch of Phillips Ltd., Hamburg, Federal Republic of Germany

Professor H. Lüthy, Riehen, Switzerland

Professor O. Mattsson, X-Ray Department, Karolinska Hospital, Stockholm, Sweden

Dr M. Nell, Laboratory for Radiological and Electromedical Testing, General Hospital of the City of Vienna, Austria

Professor L. Oliva, General Secretary, European Radiological Society, Rapallo, Italy

Professor O. Olsson, former Chief of the Department of Diagnostic Radiology, University Clinics, Lund, Sweden

Dr S. B. Osborn, St Albans, England (*representing the International Radiation Protection Association*)

Professor I. Pana, Institute of Medicine and Pharmacy, Bucharest, Romania

Dr L. Panzer, Society for Radiation and Environmental Research, Neuherberg, Federal Republic of Germany

Professor W. Penn, Institute of Diagnostic Radiology, University Clinic, Nijmegen, Netherlands

Dr G. Pohle, Section of Medical Physics, Municipal Hospital, Moabit, Berlin (West)

Dr W. S. Properzio, Division of Training and Medical Applications, Bureau of Radiological Health, Department of Health and Human Services, Rockville, MD, USA (*Rapporteur*)

Dr N. T. Racoveanu, Radiation Medicine, WHO, Geneva, Switzerland (*Secretary*)

Mr B. R. Ramsay, Shimadzu Europe GmbH, Düsseldorf, Federal Republic of Germany

Dr I. Ribka, Radiology Clinic and Polyclinic University of Munich, Federal Republic of Germany

Mr S. Savikurki, Central Hospital of the University of Helsinki, Finland

Dr W. Seelentag, Ministry of the Interior, Bonn, Federal Republic of Germany (*Co-Chairman*)

Professor F. E. Stieve, Institute for Radiation Hygiene, Federal Health Office, Neuherberg, Federal Republic of Germany (*Co-Chairman*)

Professor Y. Vorobyev, Moscow Medical Haematological Institute, Moscow, USSR
Dr F. Welde, Department of Radiophysics, Ullevaal Hospital, Oslo, Norway
Mr L. Widemann, Society for Radiation and Environmental Research, Neuherberg, Federal
   Republic of Germany
Professor J. Wojtowicz, Institute of Radiology, Poznań, Poland

WHO publications may be obtained, direct or through booksellers, from:

ALGERIA	Société Nationale d'Edition et de Diffusion, 3 bd Zirout Youcef, ALGIERS
ARGENTINA	Carlos Hirsch SRL, Florida 165, Galerias Güemes, Escritorio 453/465, BUENOS AIRES
AUSTRALIA	*Mail Order Sales:* Australian Government Publishing Service, P.O. Box 84, CANBERRA A.C.T. 2600: *or over the counter from:* Australian Government Publishing Service Bookshops *at:* 70 Alinga Street, CANBERRA CITY A.C.T. 2600; 294 Adelaide Street, BRISBANE, Queensland 4000; 347 Swanston Street, MELBOURNE, VIC 3000; 309 Pitt Street, SYDNEY, N.S.W. 2000; Mt Newman House, 200 St. George's Terrace, PERTH, WA 6000; Industry House, 12 Pirie Street, ADELAIDE, SA 5000; 156–162 Macquarie Street, HOBART, TAS 7000 — Hunter Publications, 58A Gipps Street, COLLINGWOOD, VIC 3066 — R. Hill & Son Ltd., 608 St. Kilda Road, MELBOURNE, VIC 3004; Lawson House, 10–12 Clark Street, CROW'S NEST, NSW 2065
AUSTRIA	Gerold & Co., Graben 31, 1011 VIENNA I
BANGLADESH	The WHO Programme Coordinator, G.P.O. Box 250, DACCA 5 — The Association of Voluntary Agencies, P.O. Box 5045, DACCA 5
BELGIUM	Office international de Librairie, 30 avenue Marnix, 1050 BRUSSELS — *Subscriptions to World Health only:* Jean de Lannoy, 202 avenue du Roi, 1060 BRUSSELS
BRAZIL	Biblioteca Regional de Medicina OMS/OPS, Unidade de Venda de Publicações, Caixa Postal 20.381, Vila Clementino, 04023 SÃO PAULO, S.P.
BURMA	*see* India, WHO Regional Office
CANADA	*Single and bulk copies of individual publications (not subscriptions):* Canadian Public Health Association, 1335 Carling Avenue, Suite 210, OTTAWA, Ont. K1Z 8N8. *Subscriptions: Subscription orders, accompanied by cheque made out to the* Royal Bank of Canada, Ottawa, Account World Health Organization, *should be sent to the* World Health Organization, P.O. Box 1800, Postal Station B, OTTAWA, Ont. K1P 5R5. *Correspondence concerning subscriptions should be addressed to the* World Health Organization, Distribution and Sales, 1211 GENEVA 27, Switzerland
CHINA	China National Publications Import Corporation, P.O. Box 88, BEIJING (PEKING)
COLOMBIA	Distrilibros Ltd., Pio Alfonso García, Carrera 4a, Nos 36–119, CARTAGENA
CYPRUS	Publishers' Distributors Cyprus, 30 Democratias Ave Ayios Dhometious, P.O. Box 4165, NICOSIA
CZECHO-SLOVAKIA	Artia, Ve Smeckach 30, 111 27 PRAGUE 1
DENMARK	Munksgaard Export and Subscription Service, Nørre Søgade 35, 1370 COPENHAGEN K
ECUADOR	Libreria Cientifica S.A., P.O. Box 362, Luque 223, GUAYAQUIL
EGYPT	Osiris Office for Books and Reviews, 50 Kasr El Nil Street, CAIRO
EL SALVADOR	Librería Estudiantil, Edificio Comercial B No 3, Avenida Libertad, SAN SALVADOR
FIJI	The WHO Programme Coordinator, P.O. Box 113, SUVA
FINLAND	Akateeminen Kirjakauppa, Keskuskatu 2, 00101 HELSINKI 10
FRANCE	Librairie Arnette, 2 rue Casimir-Delavigne, 75006 PARIS
GERMAN DEMOCRATIC REPUBLIC	Buchhaus Leipzig, Postfach 140, 701 LEIPZIG
GERMANY, FEDERAL REPUBLIC OF	Govi-Verlag GmbH, Ginnheimerstrasse 20, Postfach 5360, 6236 ESCHBORN — W. E. Saarbach, Postfach 101 610, Follerstrasse 2, 5000 COLOGNE 1 — Alex. Horn, Spiegelgasse 9, Postfach 3340, 6200 WIESBADEN
GHANA	Fides Enterprises, P.O. Box 1628, ACCRA
GREECE	G:C. Eleftheroudakis S.A., Librairie internationale, rue Nikis 4, ATHENS (T. 126)
HAITI	Max Bouchereau, Librairie "A la Caravelle", Boîte postale 111-B, PORT-AU-PRINCE
HONG KONG	Hong Kong Government Information Services, Beaconsfield House, 6th Floor, Queen's Road, Central, VICTORIA
HUNGARY	Kultura, P.O.B. 149, BUDAPEST 62 — Akadémiai Könyvesbolt, Váci utca 22, BUDAPEST V
ICELAND	Snaebjørn Jonsson & Co., P.O. Box 1131, Hafnarstraeti 9, REYKJAVIK
INDIA	WHO Regional Office for South-East Asia, World Health House, Indraprastha Estate, Ring Road, NEW DELHI 110002 — Oxford Book & Stationery Co., Scindia House, NEW DELHI 110001; 17 Park Street, CALCUTTA 700016 (*Sub-agent*)
INDONESIA	M/s Kalman Book Service Ltd., Kwitang Raya No. 11, P.O. Box 3105/Jkt, JAKARTA
IRAN	Iranian Amalgamated Distribution Agency, 151 Khiaban Soraya, TEHERAN
IRAQ	Ministry of Information, National House for Publishing, Distributing and Advertising, BAGHDAD
IRELAND	The Stationery Office, DUBLIN 4
ISRAEL	Heiliger & Co., 3 Nathan Strauss Street, JERUSALEM
ITALY	Edizioni Minerva Medica, Corso Bramante 83–85, 10126 TURIN; Via Lamarmora 3, 20100 MILAN
JAPAN	Maruzen Co. Ltd., P.O. Box 5050, TOKYO International, 100–31
KOREA REPUBLIC OF	The WHO Programme Coordinator, Central P.O. Box 540, SEOUL
KUWAIT	The Kuwait Bookshops Co. Ltd., Thunayan Al-Ghanem Bldg, P.O. Box 2942, KUWAIT
LAO PEOPLE'S DEMOCRATIC REPUBLIC	The WHO Programme Coordinator, P.O. Box 343, VIENTIANE
LEBANON	The Levant Distributors Co. S.A.R.L., Box 1181, Makdassi Street, Hanna Bldg, BEIRUT

WHO publications may be obtained, direct or through booksellers, from:

LUXEMBOURG	Librairie du Centre, 49 bd Royal, LUXEMBOURG
MALAWI	Malawi Book Service, P.O. Box 30044, Chichiti, BLANTYRE 3
MALAYSIA	The WHO Programme Coordinator, Room 1004, Fitzpatrick Building, Jalan Raja Chulan, KUALA LUMPUR 05–02 — Jubilee (Book) Store Ltd, 97 Jalan Tuanku Abdul Rahman, P.O. Box 629, KUALA LUMPUR 01–08 — Parry's Book Center, K. L. Hilton Hotel, Jln. Treacher, P.O. Box 960, KUALA LUMPUR
MEXICO	La Prensa Médica Mexicana, Ediciones Científicas, Paseo de las Facultades 26, Apt. Postal 20–413, MEXICO CITY 20, D.F.
MONGOLIA	see India, WHO Regional Office
MOROCCO	Editions La Porte, 281 avenue Mohammed V, RABAT
MOZAMBIQUE	INLD, Caixa Postal 4030, MAPUTO
NEPAL	see India, WHO Regional Office
NETHERLANDS	Medical Books Europe BV, Noorderwal 38, 7241 BL LOCHEM
NEW ZEALAND	Government Printing Office, Publications Section, Mulgrave Street, Private Bag, WELLINGTON 1; Walter Street, WELLINGTON; World Trade Building, Cubacade, Cuba Street, WELLINGTON. *Government Bookshops at:* Hannaford Burton Building, Rutland Street, Private Bag, AUCKLAND; 159 Hereford Street, Private Bag, CHRISTCHURCH; Alexandra Street, P.O. Box 857, HAMILTON; T & G Building, Princes Street, P.O. Box 1104, DUNEDIN — R. Hill & Son Ltd, Ideal House, Cnr Gillies Avenue & Eden Street, Newmarket, AUCKLAND 1
NIGERIA	University Bookshop Nigeria Ltd, University of Ibadan, IBADAN
NORWAY	J. G. Tanum A/S, P.O. Box 1177 Sentrum, OSLO 1
PAKISTAN	Mirza Book Agency, 65 Shahrah–E–Quaid–E–Azam, P.O. Box 729, LAHORE 3
PAPUA NEW GUINEA	The WHO Programme Coordinator, P.O. Box 5896, BOROKO
PHILIPPINES	World Health Organization, Regional Office for the Western Pacific, P.O. Box 2932, MANILA — The Modern Book Company Inc., P.O. Box 632, 922 Rizal Avenue, MANILA 2800
POLAND	Składnica Księgarska, ul Mazowiecka 9, 00052 WARSAW *(except periodicals)* — BKWZ Ruch, ul Wronia 23, 00840 WARSAW *(periodicals only)*
PORTUGAL	Livraria Rodrigues, 186 Rua do Ouro, LISBON 2
SIERRA LEONE	Njala University College Bookshop (University of Sierra Leone), Private Mail Bag, FREETOWN
SINGAPORE	The WHO Programme Coordinator, 144 Moulmein Road, G.P.O. Box 3457, SINGAPORE 1 — Select Books (Pte) Ltd, 215 Tanglin Shopping Centre, 2/F, 19 Tanglin Road, SINGAPORE 10
SOUTH AFRICA	Van Schaik's Bookstore (Pty) Ltd, P.O. Box 724, 268 Church Street, PRETORIA 0001
SPAIN	Comercial Atheneum S.A., Consejo de Ciento 130–136, BARCELONA 15; General Moscardó 29, MADRID 20 — Librería Díaz de Santos, Lagasca 95 y Maldonado 6, MADRID 6; Balmes 417 y 419, BARCELONA 22
SRI LANKA	see India, WHO Regional Office
SWEDEN	Aktiebolaget C.E. Fritzes Kungl. Hovbokhandel, Regeringsgatan 12, 10327 STOCKHOLM
SWITZERLAND	Medizinischer Verlag Hans Huber, Länggass Strasse 76, 3012 BERNE 9
SYRIAN ARAB REPUBLIC	M. Farras Kekhia, P.O. Box No. 5221, ALEPPO
THAILAND	see India, WHO Regional Office
TUNISIA	Société Tunisienne de Diffusion, 5 avenue de Carthage, TUNIS
TURKEY	Haset Kitapevi, 469 Istiklal Caddesi, Beyoglu, ISTANBUL
UNITED KINGDOM	H.M. Stationery Office: 49 High Holborn, LONDON WC1V 6HB; 13a Castle Street, EDINBURGH EH2 3AR; 41 The Hayes, CARDIFF CF1 1JW; 80 Chichester Street, BELFAST BT1 4JY; Brazennose Street, MANCHESTER M60 8AS; 258 Broad Street, BIRMINGHAM B1 2HE; Southey House, Wine Street, BRISTOL BS1 2BQ. *All mail orders should be sent to* P.O. Box 569, LONDON SE1 9NH
UNITED STATES OF AMERICA	*Single and bulk copies of individual publications (not subscriptions):* WHO Publications Centre USA, 49 Sheridan Avenue, ALBANY, N.Y. 12210. *Subscriptions: Subscription orders, accompanied by check made out to the* Chemical Bank, New York, Account World Health Organization, *should be sent to the* World Health Organization, P.O. Box 5284, Church Street Station, NEW YORK, N.Y. 10249: *Correspondence concerning subscriptions should be addressed to the* World Health Organization, Distribution and Sales, 1211 GENEVA 27, Switzerland. *Publications are also available from the* United Nations Bookshop, NEW YORK, N.Y. 10017 *(retail only)*
USSR	*For readers in the USSR requiring Russian editions:* Komsomolskij prospekt 18, Medicinskaja Kniga, Moscow — *For readers outside the USSR requiring Russian editions:* ...izneckij most 18, Meždunarodnaja Kniga, MOSCOW G-200
VENEZUELA	Editorial Interamericana de Venezuela C.A., Apartado 50.785, CARACAS 105 — Librería del Este, Apartado 60.337, CARACAS 106 — Librería Médica Paris, Apartado 60.681, CARACAS 106
YUGOSLAVIA	Jugoslovenska Knjiga, Terazije 27/II, 11000 BELGRADE
ZAIRE	Librairie universitaire, avenue de la Paix Nº 167, B.P. 1682, KINSHASA I

Special terms for developing countries are obtainable on application to the WHO Programme Coordinators or WHO Regional Offices listed above or to the World Health Organization, Distribution and Sales Service, 1211 Geneva 27, Switzerland. Orders from countries where sales agents have not yet been appointed may also be sent to the Geneva address, but must be paid for in pounds sterling, US dollars, or Swiss francs.

Price: Sw. fr.11 —   Prices are subject to change without notice.